D0429110

THE
HOT
DIET

THE HOT DIET

THE <u>REAL</u> REASON YOU'RE
GAINING WEIGHT . . . AND HOW TO
LOSE IT FAST AND FOREVER

AJ Djo

with Bill Quinn

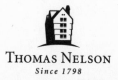

THOMAS NELSON
Since 1798

NASHVILLE   DALLAS   MEXICO CITY   RIO DE JANEIRO   BEIJING

Copyright © 2006 by Ali Djowharzadeh

The Hot Diet provides information of a general nature, and readers are strongly cautioned to consult with a physician or other healthcare professional before engaging in any of the programs described herein. This book is not to be used as an alternative method for conditions requiring the services of a personal physician.

Information contained in this book or in any other publication, article, Web site, etc. should not be considered a substitute for consultation with a board-certified doctor to address individual medical needs. Individual facts and circumstances will determine the treatment that is most appropriate. *The Hot Diet* Publisher and its Authors, AJ Djo and Bill Quinn, disclaim any liability, loss, or damage that might result in the implementation of the contents of this book.

All rights reserved. No portion of this book may be reproduced, stored in a retrieval system, or transmitted in any form or by any means—electronic, mechanical, photocopy, recording, scanning, or other—except for brief quotations in critical reviews or articles, without the prior written permission of the publisher.

Published in Nashville, TN, by Thomas Nelson. Thomas Nelson is a trademark of Thomas Nelson, Inc.

Thomas Nelson, Inc. titles may be purchased in bulk for educational, business, fund-raising, or sales promotional use. For information, please e-mail SpecialMarkets@ThomasNelson.com.

Library of Congress Cataloging-in-Publication Data

Djo, AJ, 1953–
  The hot diet : the real reason you're gaining weight—and how to lose it fast and forever / AJ Djo with Bill Quinn.
      p. cm.
  ISBN-13: 978-0-7852-2219-4 (hardcover)
  ISBN-10: 0-7852-2219-7
  1. Weight loss. 2. Reducing diets. 3. Refrigerated foods. I. Quinn,
Bill, 1946– II. Title.
RM222.2.D594 2006
613.2'5—dc22

                                                              2006100090

Printed in the United States of America
07 08 09 10 11 **QWM** 6 5 4 3 2 1

Indebtedness and praise to the One
who has given us the gift of life.

May the Creator of soul and body
be honored and glorified as we fulfill
our obligation to care for, nourish,
and protect our amazing bodies.

To Jenn,
Wish you health, wealth
& Blissful life,

AJ DJ

8-15-17

CONTENTS

1: THE POISON

Something is killing millions of Americans, and as I write this, I am less than two days from finding out what it is.

It's not any of the reasons touted by the popular diet books—not about carbohydrates versus proteins, food zones, or the right carbs versus wrong carbs, nor is it about about weighing every morsel or counting every calorie. What's making you and me overweight cannot be fixed by a magic new drug or supplement.

Instead, it's a deadly poison guaranteed to be on your breakfast, lunch, or dinner table this very day. Eliminate this poison, and you can kiss your weight problems goodbye. Can you imagine more important news than the key to ending decades of diet wars?

As a reader of this book, you are about to discover for the first time in your life why you keep adding pounds year after year. Of course, I'm assuming you're overweight and want your trim body back. You want to recapture the energy you used to have, and you'll do almost anything to recover it. But even if you're not overweight, the secrets you're about to learn could ensure that you never will be.

———————————

It's been almost a week now since my first meeting with the man whose card read "AJ Djo."

"Nobody can pronounce my last name," he had warned me in advance. "Call me AJ."

I arrived at the restaurant early for our lunch meeting, looking expectantly at each stranger walking through the door of the waiting area to see if it was AJ. Then I saw a man walk in with a bright smile and sparkling eyes. He was trim, appeared to be in excellent shape, and his demeanor was warm and welcoming. There was an unusual energy about this man that immediately captured my attention.

"Bill, I have so much to tell you."

"I'm all ears, AJ. But let's order first."

AJ had set our meeting to discuss what he called an incredible new breakthrough in dieting. As we ordered, I watched him for clues. I had my usual hamburger and diet cola. Surprisingly, he ordered a hamburger as well, replacing the cola with water.

Was cola the culprit?

"No, no," he laughed. "I just feel like a burger and water today."

After some small talk, AJ told me his story:

— I GRADUATED FROM THE UNIVERSITY OF OKLAHOMA TWENTY-some years ago, first studying premed for three years before switching over to chemical engineering. I worked my way through school selling books door-to-door for Thomas Nelson Publishing.

It was then, less than five minutes into our conversation, that I discovered AJ's love for storytelling.

— YOU WANT TO LEARN ABOUT PEOPLE? TRY SELLING BOOKS door-to-door. Once you get past the natural barriers that people put up against door-to-door salesmen, you discover how good people really are. Most of the time, once I got people talking, I just sat back and observed. You'd be surprised what you learn.

For example, I knocked on the door of a home in a small town in North Carolina, and a little old blue-haired lady came to the door carrying a shotgun. Startled, I started to retreat down the sidewalk.

"C'mon back here, young fellow. What you selling there?"

Summoning my courage and with a wary eye on the shotgun, I nervously started my pitch. It turned out the lady was unusually friendly and full of Southern charm, which didn't explain the gun now leaning up against the rocker beside her. A few minutes later, the lady was writing a check. I asked her why, as an apparently peace-loving person, she carried the gun.

"I always give folks a chance to prove themselves," she

replied. "If they talk like they belong to Jesus, I give Jesus back to them. If they don't, I give them the buckshot!"

Treat others as they treat you, the lady was suggesting. It was a lesson I have never forgotten.

Leaning forward earnestly, AJ finally got down to business.

"Bill, I want to tell you why I called this meeting and how I made an incredible discovery about health and dieting."

Finally, the good stuff, I thought. I signaled the waitress for another cola.

AJ told me that after graduation he had found an entry-level position in chemical engineering. He soon rose through the ranks to become a successful consultant in the quickly growing field of semiconductors. His ability to solve problems through the powers of observation brought him great financial success. As his reputation grew, companies around the world began demanding his attention. His travels took him all over the U.S., Europe, and Asia, allowing him to rub shoulders with the Pope, dine with presidents of companies and countries, and work intimately with some of the largest companies in the world.

"One day I even had dinner with Ronald Reagan," he said proudly.

"You did? And Reagan taught you about dieting?"

"No, no." He laughed. "But if you listen closely, you might spot some clues."

— It was 1977, at a function in the future president's honor, and I found myself sitting across from Reagan. I was immediately captivated by his intelligence and wit, mostly listening, when Reagan suddenly leaned across the table and asked me about my plans for the future. I told him I'd always dreamed of living in California one day.

Reagan smiled brightly. "I hope you do go to California one day, AJ. It's a beautiful state, part of a beautiful country, part of this beautiful planet we live on. We all should strive to leave it a better place than we found it. A simple test is to ask yourself: Do you want people to say it's a better place because he lived here or because he left it?"

Reagan then launched into a story about an immigrant who traveled to California carrying nothing but a single suitcase. Ten years later, he owned several buildings and businesses. When an admirer asked the immigrant what was in the suitcase, he said, "Two million in cash and one million in notes!" Reagan led the laughter that erupted up and down the table.

Then when the food arrived, I noticed something interesting, especially for a politician—or my idea of what politicians are like.

Reagan paused a moment as though in private prayer, much like a singer pauses before starting a song. It was as if he was being respectful to the food, which he then began to eat slowly and quietly. I was struck by his peacefulness, almost as if he was in a spiritual state.

After the meal, Reagan drank a warm beverage. Noticing that he was about to go to the podium for his speech, I reached over to shake his hand. I was struck by how strong and rough it was. I asked him if by chance he enjoyed gardening as George Washington had.

Reagan looked a bit startled but smiled at the comparison. Then I blurted out that I hoped he'd run for president in 1980 and that I thought he would definitely win and become a great president like Washington because they were both wise and accomplished listeners.

As AJ finished his story, I tried to dig out the clue he had said might be there.

"So the secret to successful dieting is to—what?—be calm during meals and be a good listener? That's it?"

"That's part of it, Bill. But the core secret is something else."

I urged AJ to continue.

— MY SUCCESS AS A CHEMICAL ENGINEER GREW YEAR AFTER year. But in early 2000, a dark cloud entered my tidy little world.

One day I noticed that my son, John, was getting a bit pudgy around the waist. Not only that, but the boy was spending more and more time slumped in a chair playing video games. While other kids were out running and playing, John was in his room staring at the screen.

"John, you need to get out and get some exercise. Turn off that worthless game!"

"Aw, Dad, there's nothing wrong with video games. All the kids play video games."

But I was undeterred. My son's expanding waist and lethargy could not be healthy. In fact, looking down at my own generous waistline, I wondered if my son was not the only one with a problem.

What was causing John to gain excess pounds? Knowing it

was my responsibility, I took the initiative and had John cut back on the games and started him on a fitness program. But his weight gain continued.

My concern for John eventually led me on a five-year investigation into America's problem with obesity. Using the same scientific methods and observational skills that had brought me success in the business world, I began to observe people in every conceivable dining situation. I watched people in fine restaurants, in fast-food establishments, at the mall, and in their homes.

"See that young lady at the table over there, Bill? Notice anything about her?"

I followed his eyes and looked at the woman, perhaps twenty years old, sipping a drink and picking at her salad. She looked normal to me, maybe a few pounds overweight.

"Beats me."

AJ then described how he had observed more than 104,000 people eating much the same as the young woman at the next table.

— I HAD FILLED DOZENS OF BULGING NOTEBOOKS WITH RECORD-ings of what people ate and drank, in what proportions, and in what combinations. I had recorded who was overweight and who was not. Then I tried boiling down all that data, looking for a connection. But the answer eluded me.

Surprisingly, I observed that people eating the same foods in similar quantities could be a perfectly normal weight *or* obese.

"Look at the couple over there," he suggested, motioning to the middle-aged couple to our left. "They're both having salads and steak. Yet the husband looks as if he's about forty pounds overweight, and the wife looks just about right. Why is that?"

I shrugged my shoulders. I'd seen a million couples like that.

"The clue is right there in front of your eyes, Bill. Do you see it?"

I looked again very intently. But for the life of me, I saw nothing.

"There's a clue there?"

"Yes," AJ smiled, "right before your eyes."

He then asked if I remembered the FedEx logo.

"The red and white one? Sure. FedEx comes by my office all the time. In fact, I have a sign I hang in the window when I need a pickup."

"Have you ever noticed the arrow in that logo?"

"FedEx has an arrow in its logo? You're sure?"

"Check it out. Next time you see a FedEx truck, look for the arrow in the logo. You'd be surprised," he said, glancing over at the couple, "at the things we look at and never actually see. Once you notice the arrow, you'll never miss it again."

Continuing the story of his research, he told me about the many studies showing that Americans today are much heavier than just thirty years ago. What had changed? What had been added to the American diet that was not present several decades ago?

As his business took him to other countries, he noticed that obesity was nowhere as prevalent as it was in the United States.

—I PERSONALLY OBSERVED THE FRENCH, ITALIANS, JAPANESE, and many others in my travels. Most of them were at recommended weight levels. Yet these same people move to the United States, and it's not long before they're as overweight as the rest of us. Then I began to hear reports that even in foreign countries the incidence of obesity was beginning to increase. It's like they're a decade behind us with this problem. Whatever is affecting Americans was starting to affect them too.

Was the whole world suffering an obesity epidemic with the U.S. among the first to be affected? What was causing this epidemic? Was it something in our food? Was it a chemical reaction? Were so-called diet gurus correct in saying we were simply eating too much protein or too many carbohydrates?

Or was it something far more sinister?

At one point I found myself wondering if hostile governments were deliberately putting something into our food. What better way to bring down America than by making its people lazy and obese, overloading its economic system with billions of dollars in medical bills, lost wages, and lost man-hours? Perhaps I'd been watching too many bad movies.

Then one day, when I least expected it, my search came to an end. I was relaxing on the patio, enjoying the sunny weather. Soon the temperatures started to climb, so I was thankful when my wife brought out a tall glass of iced tea. As always, as I leaned back in the lounge, my mind wandered to my quest. Slowly stirring the tea, listening to the gentle chimes of the ice cubes clinking against the frosty glass, I again asked the questions that had plagued me for more than five years now: *Why are Americans getting so heavy? What are we doing now that we were not doing thirty or forty years ago? Why have people from other nations been so much thinner until just recently? Is there a poison in our diets?*

And suddenly, there it was.

After years of searching, the answer was right in front of me. In a moment of earth-shaking illumination, I knew why Americans were so overweight. I knew why two people could eat almost identical foods and one would gain weight while the other would not, why the problem was only recently beginning to show up in other countries, and how obesity—if not checked—would soon hold the entire world in its grasp. The culprit was so innocent in appearance, so accepted, so omni-present, that it almost made me question my own findings. But thinking back to bits of suddenly linked data in my massive research materials, I realized it was dead-on.

America was eating herself to death, and I knew why.

Running for my notebooks, I dug into pages crammed with thousands of observations, revisiting instance after instance where I had noted exactly who was eating and drinking what, and whether they were heavy or not.

In case after case, "it" was as clear as the arrow in the FedEx logo.

Immediately I knew I had to tell someone. I had to tell the whole world. Remembering that my neighbor was a magazine publisher, I called to see if he could recommend a writer for this scientist with a story to tell. That's how Bill and I came to have our first lunch together.

That first meeting with AJ lasted more than two hours. As he spoke, I found myself wrestling with the possibility that this quiet, unassuming man before me had solved one of society's most challenging puzzles. Could he have discovered the key to avoiding obesity? But he wouldn't disclose the details.

"I'll tell you what the poison is, but in due time."

By now the waitress had cleared away our dishes, and I was on my third cola. Closing my jacket over my own expanding waistline, I asked him if America's fixation with diet fads was a contributing factor. After all, the last thing we need is another diet.

"You're right, we don't need another diet. We just need a diet that works. The fact that the bookstores are filled with diet books just means that no one has found the right answer yet."

"Makes sense. So you know beyond a doubt why these other diets don't work?"

"Oh, a few of them seem to work at first, but none of them work long term. If they did, we wouldn't be buying new diet books all the time. Millions of people start these diets, but a few months later, they fall off the wagon and back into their old habits. How many diet books do you have in your house, Bill?"

"I lost count."

"Exactly. I concluded that some fad diets have elements that work and other elements that do not. Most diets are downright boring. They say you have to sacrifice many of your favorite foods in order to lose weight."

"Last time I dieted, AJ, I sure got tired of eating meat night after night—with no bread or potatoes."

"Millions of other Americans are tired, too, Bill. But suppose

I could show you a diet that really isn't a diet at all? It's a completely natural solution to your dieting problems. Even more than that, it's a lifestyle you can easily and enthusiastically follow the rest of your life. You'll no longer have a weight problem, you won't be hungry, and you'll have more energy than you ever imagined possible. All because my diet has the breakthrough discovery the others lack."

"And you're not going to tell me what it is?"

"Not yet. First I'd like you to try this new diet for yourself. I'm going to give you a seven-day plan," he said, pulling out some sheets of paper, "that will give you a small foretaste of what it can do for you."

"OK, AJ, but I don't mind telling you I'm a bit skeptical. Remember, I tried high-protein/low-carb diets, and I don't know how many others. Yet I still gained back the pounds. But what have I got to lose?"

"Maybe as much as three or more pounds a week, Bill. Actually, it's good you're skeptical. All our lives people come up with new things and ask us to believe in them. If you can experience something, then you can be a true believer. You will feel very little hunger on this plan, and you will not deny yourself any important fruits, vegetables, or even bread. You must promise to eat or drink only what is in this plan. I have, however, included some substitute foods in case you don't like a particular item."

"Fair enough."

"Also, I want you to do some light research for your own benefit. Look at what's happening with weight in America. Read up on how obesity is making huge changes in our nation. Look over the diets being promoted at the local bookstores, and see if you can spot why most people soon give up on them. Find out what you can, and then we can talk."

"Lunch a week from today, same time and place?"

"Agreed. And one last thing, Bill. Promise me you'll take a walk every day. At least fifteen minutes long, but thirty minutes if you can."

"Do I absolutely have to exercise?"

"Beyond question. You know why so many people hate to exercise?"

"We're lazy?"

"No, we just don't have the energy. I heard that countless times over the past five years. With this diet, you will have all the energy you want, more than you've had in a long time."

Suddenly I knew my days as a couch bunny were numbered. "OK, if I can coax my oversized carcass into forward motion, I'll do the walking too."

"Bill, you'll thank me for this. I promise you. When I tell you the secret, you'll be blown away."

With that, I ended my first meeting with the man who believes he can save the lives of millions of people worldwide. I had learned just enough to be intrigued.

Thankfully, he had not attacked me for what I ordered for lunch.

Obesity is not directly related to whether you had fries with your burger at lunch today although you'd be wise to do without them. They're full of empty calories that do you and your cholesterol count no good. Obesity is not a direct result of something as simple as how much protein or carbohydrate is in your diet. So unless you've got some kind of medical condition, you can no longer blame your thunderous thighs and pendulous tummy on the usual suspects suggested by "experts" who don't know what they're talking about.

You can imagine the questions I had. What "poison" had AJ discovered? Was it some chemical in the water we drink? Too much meat or not enough grain or fiber? Or was it something far-out like the aluminum in our coke cans? Was it the smog in the air?

AJ had said it's nothing I would have guessed—that it's something incredibly simple.

"Be patient." The most important discovery of the century and he wanted to wait another week to tell me? Arriving home, I was frustrated, so I grabbed some leftover chicken salad from the fridge and washed it down with some iced tea. *Hmmm, a chemical engineer who's discovered the diet breakthrough of the century*, I thought as I sucked on an ice cube. *Bet you a dime to a dollar, it's sugar. Yeah, gotta be the sugar.*

I began to research the problem as AJ had suggested.

A government report entitled the 2003–2004 National Health and Nutrition Examination Survey (NHANES) found that two out of three Americans are either overweight or obese.[1] That was news to me. *Two out of three?* Then I thought back to the last time I was in an airport, passing the time while waiting for my flight, engaging in a little people watching. So it wasn't my imagination, after all—there were more overweight people than there used to be.

The International Food Information Council Foundation

on Obesity and Weight Management reported that approximately 400,000 people die each year because of poor diet and lack of exercise.[2]

In addition to the huge emotional cost of so many premature deaths, there is also a financial cost. Research data shows that medical treatment costs resulting from overweight and obesity accounted for over 90 billion dollars of U.S. health and related medical expenditures.[3]

This was far more serious than I had ever dreamed. How had the problem become so serious? What was happening to us?

It got worse. The next day an online article showed more fallout from the problem. Life expectancy in the U.S., it read, will fall dramatically in the near future due to obesity.[4] This was a significant shift from previous predictions of increasingly longer life spans.

According to the article, within fifty years obesity will reduce the average life span of 77.6 years by at least two to five years.[5] Not good news when you consider that the life expectancy of Americans already lags behind that of twenty other developed countries.[6]

Even if someone is not overweight now, there's likely an overweight or even obese version of him or her in the future. Not only is the United States one of the most obese societies in the world, but imagine what we'll be like twenty years from now.

If obesity increases, so will the diseases related to it. Hospital and medical costs could skyrocket just when Baby Boomers are settling down to retirement. Soon we could have more people living on retirement income, with more medical problems and higher medical bills than ever before in history.

How's that for a retirement scenario?

Not only that, but AJ's son can expect lots of company if his weight problem continues. Numerous studies are now showing a huge increase in the number of children who are overweight or obese. Think back to when you were a child. Thirty years ago, overweight and obese children were relatively rare. The grade school in which I grew up may have had two or three overweight kids out of a couple of hundred students. I remember a few instances of kids being called "fat," but those were few and far between.

Not so in today's schools.

Between 1963 and 1970, just 4 percent of children in schools were overweight, according to data from the National Health and Nutrition Examination Survey. In the 1999–2002 survey period, that number had risen to 15.8 percent.[7]

What's happening to our children? What are we doing to them that could potentially threaten their futures? How many billions of dollars will be spent one day in medical bills for weight-related diseases such as diabetes, cancer, and heart attacks?

It's even worse with adults. More and more adults gain unwanted pounds every year. Talk with virtually anyone, and either that person or someone close to him has a weight problem. What does the future hold for a nation in which most of its citizens are overweight, are being treated for obesity-related diseases, or who simply lack the energy to face the challenging tasks that made us great? Will we go down in history as the *fat nation*?

The full impact of what AJ had shared with me was starting to hit home.

AJ's diet discovery could not only change your understanding of why you add on pounds over the years, but it could dramatically alter the kind of person you are—for the better. It could change not only your weight but also your outlook on life. You can once again be the trim, healthy, energetic person you remember from your high school yearbooks or wedding photos (go even further back than that, if you have to).

Before you finish reading this book, AJ's breakthrough discovery will show you how. In our next meeting, AJ promised to reveal a simple truth that has eluded man throughout the past century.

In the Middle Ages, obesity was actually regarded favorably, indicating a person who was well fed. It was not by accident that in the 1600s artist Peter Paul Rubens painted women with voluminous bodies. It was exactly what his audience wanted to see. Back then, people admired heavier figures and equated excess weight with excess money for food. If you were fat, you were wealthy.

Funny how that interpretation has changed. Granted, some men still prefer heavier women. But for the majority, thin is in. Thin is on fashion runways. It's at the malls. Unfortunately, it's not in the person staring sadly at us from our mirrors every morning. Most of us are either well on our way to becoming as fat as Rubens's models, or we've already arrived.

As I waited for my meeting with AJ, wondering what the secret might be, my mind wandered back to my own struggles with weight. As a youngster growing up in a small farming community in southern Wisconsin, I was surrounded by all kinds of dairy products, homemade pies and desserts, steaming hot homemade bread fresh from Mom's oven, and all the red meat I could eat. We broke just about every diet rule you can think of, yet my eight siblings and I were so skinny and wiry that Mom actually worried about us.

"Have some seconds," she would say, "so the neighbors don't think we're abusing you kids by starving you to death."

What changed from those days to now? We were an average family (other than the fact that we could field our own baseball team—and did), eating the typical home-cooked American diet of bread, red meat, potatoes, veggies, and cheese casseroles. Why weren't we obese as children?

"The answer is right under your nose," AJ had told me. "It's a poison you consume with virtually every meal."

For most of my life, my weight was right where the weight charts said it should be. I was usually trim, but if occasionally a slight bulge occurred around my waist and betrayed short periods of indulgence, I could diet it away in a couple of weeks or so. Then one day a terrible thing happened.

I turned forty.

Suddenly, it became harder and harder to lose those bulges. I found myself wearing larger pant sizes and longer belts. I no longer played weekly tennis at 6:00 a.m. on Fridays, was too tired to run three miles a day, and had less and less time to shoot buckets with the guys on Saturday mornings. I was getting around less and getting ever larger.

You could see the difference inside my closet.

Over the years, I found myself with two sizes of clothing: "normal" and "large." As my weight changed, so did the clothes I fit into. At any given time, I could wear only half of my wardrobe, saving the other half for when my weight changed. That meant I could never get rid of either group.

Imagine how much space could be saved all across America if closets were suddenly emptied of all the clothes people can no longer fit into. We'd have walk-in closets we could actually walk inside. *His* and *her* closets would become *ours* again. On second thought, that might not be such a good idea. As a husband, I never got my fair share of the territory when my wife and I used the same closet. The fact that I had three pairs of shoes to her fifty and four suits to her twenty may have had something to do with it.

If you want your marriage to last, never share the same closet with your spouse.

In any event, by the time I was fifty, my large clothes had become normal, and I had added a new size called *larger still*.

What I didn't know was that I was in step with much of the rest of America. After the age of thirty, the average American starts adding ugly pounds and inches. Some attribute this to our tendency to exercise less after age thirty. Others blame it on slowing metabolism, contending that metabolism can slow as much as 1 percent a year once we hit our thirties.[8] Was this what AJ's discovery was all about? Had he found the answer to why we gain weight as we age?

As my stomach gradually pushed my belt to the last hole and eventually sloped well beyond it, I chased every diet program that came down the pike. I followed the Pritikin diet, the Atkins diet, the Zone, and others.

I never tried the South Beach Diet. It sounded too much like the Atkins diet to gain my interest.

To be honest, I lost weight with most of the diets I tried. Sometimes I even lost a lot of weight, but it always came back. Among my more recent attempts was the Atkins diet—twice. The first time on the diet I lost twenty-three pounds, which was fantastic and made me feel on top of the world again. But after four months of high protein meals, I was bored. I felt that if I didn't eat some carbs soon, I was going to go ballistic. So I jumped off the meat wagon and soothed my carb-starved body with bread, potatoes, fruit, and dairy products—all the things that Atkins had limited. Not only did the food taste better, but I comforted myself by listening to Atkins critics who claimed the diet was endangering my health. Of course, the pounds came back.

A few months later, I gave the Atkins diet another try. This time I lost thirteen pounds in three weeks. Yet once again I grew so tired of eating meat and eggs that I soon dropped it.

Not long after that—with a big, carb-engorged sandwich in one hand and a frosty mug of soda in the other—I was congratulating myself on getting back to a "real" diet. Sure, the bathroom scale creaked with the increasing load each morning, but I felt safer not worrying about what too much meat might be doing to my arteries.

I had lots of company. Most of the people I knew were on diets. In fact, we change diets more often than some people change socks. Any weight we lose on a diet, we gain back—plus a couple of pounds extra. Sound familiar?

All that is about to change, AJ had promised me. Yo-yo dieting does not have to be a way of life. We can return to our trimmer, more energetic selves. No matter how many times we have tried, no matter how often we have failed, there's a new and healthier way to balance our lifestyles, our weight, and our peace of mind.

The answer, he had said again and again, is everywhere we go. And just as you once discovered the arrow in the FedEx logo and will never miss it again, so you will easily and naturally incorporate this new approach to eating into your personal life.

"I'll show you why fad diets inevitably fail," AJ had promised. "Different as they are, they share the same fatal flaw. America is on a diet merry-go-round, and these countless fads are not only making us dizzy but making the problem worse."

What would you give to know the secret that will end your weight-gain problems forever? What would you give to be thin without starving yourself, without feeling deprived, without restricting favorite foods, without any limits at all—except one?

Your family will be happier. Your friends and fellow workers will be happier. But most importantly, you will be happier.

What is this diet breakthrough that AJ has discovered? Is it everything he says it is?

Five days into the new diet he gave me, I lost four pounds. It could have been my imagination, but my belt seemed just a bit less tight. I had more energy than I'd experienced in a long time. I looked forward to my walks. In the evenings, I found myself getting up off the couch, turning off the TV, and looking for physical things to do. I even pulled my dusty set of free weights out of the storage cabinet in the garage.

I was doing all this without hunger pangs, with no worries

about how too many or too few carbs or proteins might be damaging my health, without giving up fruits or vegetables, with no feeling of deprivation at all. In fact, I felt better after these meals than I had in a long time.

2: THE QUEST

"Order anything you want," AJ said, smiling broadly.
At long last, my second meeting with AJ had arrived. I could hardly wait to get the details.

"I'll just have some soup and salad, and maybe a cola," I said to the waitress. The seven-day diet AJ had given me was now over, and I didn't want to jeopardize the weight I had lost—now totaling a respectable five pounds. I wasn't sure what the "poison" was that AJ had warned me about. He had not told me what he was taking out of my diet that was so terrible, and for the life of me, I had not been able to figure it out. Now, at our second meal together, I was more than a little worried about embarrassing myself by ordering the "forbidden fruit" in front of him. Soup and salad should be a safe bet, I figured.

As he had done the week before, AJ ordered the same food I did.

So far, so good.

I took a long drink of cola. "Ahhhh, that hits the spot."

AJ smiled slightly. "Bill, have you ever noticed how we sometimes mistake the body's thirst as hunger?"

"No. What do you mean?"

"When the body is dehydrated, people often think they need to eat and automatically reach for a cold drink."

"And those drinks are loaded with sugar!" I said. "So is sugar the poison you talked about?"

"No, sugar is not the poison," he responded. "Sugar is, however, very addictive. The more of it you eat, the more your body craves it. The average American eats more than fifteen tablespoons of sugar per day."

"I don't ever eat sugar," I injected.

"Sure you do. How about when you have salad dressing, or crackers, or soft drinks? Consuming too much sugar has been directly related to heart disease, cancer, bone diseases, diabetes, and more."

"Well, how about salt? Is that the poison?"

"That's what a lot of people would guess, but they're wrong. We need about a fourth of a teaspoon of salt per day, about 500 mg, but the average American consumes more than ten times as much. That contributes to problems with high blood pressure, heart disease, and kidney ailments."

"AJ, I don't even touch the salt shaker. I never add salt to my food."

"But what about all the sodium in the processed and packaged foods you eat? Or what about the sodium in meats such as salami, ham, and sausage? Or cereals? Or many table condiments? Salt is all around us, and it is definitely having an impact upon our health."

He paused.

"Salt may be contributing to the health problems of some Americans, but it is not the poison I am talking about."

The suspense was getting to me. "AJ, if it's not sugar and not salt, what is it? Can we get down to brass tacks? What's making us fatter and fatter year after year?"

Since cola was apparently off the list of suspected causes, I gulped down another quick mouthful, and now that the salad had arrived served on a refreshingly frosty plate, I shoveled in a couple of mouthfuls of that as well. The cold lettuce felt good.

"Slow down, Bill," AJ said. "I see you're a fast eater. You've always been that way, right?"

I could see that AJ had me pegged. I'd been a speed eater all my life. When you grow up with eight hungry brothers and sisters, including two particularly sneaky older brothers with unnaturally sharp elbows pushing you aside at the feeding trough, you learned to eat fast or starve.

"A fast eater? Sure, I've been called that once or twice. Is that the problem? People are dying because they eat too fast?"

"No, no." He chuckled. "That's not the problem, though eating too fast certainly doesn't help your digestion much. I've just never seen someone wolf down a salad as fast as you do."

He wasn't complimenting me. I was sure of that.

"Bill, let's get down to my story. I promised to tell you the secret today. But settle back. I have a lot to tell you.

— OBESITY HAD NEVER BEEN A FACTOR IN MY LIFE UNTIL THE day I noticed my son's increasing weight and then my own expanding waistline. Shortly after that, I happened to have lunch with a long-time friend, an old college chum. Gary and I hadn't talked in almost six months, so I was looking forward to the occasion. We had barely sat down and ordered when the waitress brought a basket filled with an aromatic hot loaf of bread.

"Nice and hot. Grab a piece."

To my surprise, Gary put the basket aside. "I can't have any."

"I thought you loved bread."

"I do, AJ, but I'm on the Atkins diet and have to watch my carbs."

"I thought you were avoiding fat and counting calories."

"That was my previous diet," Gary said, a wan smile on his face. "Dr. Atkins says carbs turn into insulin, which turns into fat. So if you want to lose weight, you have to cut carbs."

Then he brightened up. "I've already lost five pounds."

"Where do carbs come from?" I asked.

"Bread, pasta, rice, potatoes, desserts, cereal, milk, fruits—"

"I thought those were good for you."

"Not anymore. If you want to lose weight, Dr. Atkins says you should avoid carbs."

I took another bite of the warm bread. Somehow it didn't taste as good as it had a moment before, and a twinge of guilt nagged at the back of my mind. The waitress approached with our order.

"No bread with your hamburger?" I noticed.

"Nope. The first couple of weeks on the Atkins diet you eat

hardly any carbs at all. I don't drink cola anymore, either, just iced tea and ice water."

"So I shouldn't have ordered the Pepsi?" The guilt was coming on again.

"Not if you want to lose weight. I need to lose twenty-five pounds, and my wife wants to lose even more. Those were our New Year's resolutions. What were yours?"

"Oh, three things: make more money, lose twenty pounds, and spend more time with the family," I said as I leaned back in my chair.

"How you doing?"

"Not so good." I laughed. "I'm making less money than last year, getting fatter, and I don't have time to even turn around!"

A serious look came over Gary's face. "AJ, you've got to get a grip on this weight thing, otherwise you're going to become obese. Did you know that two out of three Americans are classified as overweight, and one out of three is actually obese?"

"That would make it, what, 100 million obese Americans?"

"Exactly," Gary answered. "All from eating too many carbs. Rice, bread, pasta."

"That's hard to believe. People all around the world are eating tons of rice, bread, and pasta every day, and they never grow fat. Their diets are drenching with carbs!" I noted.

"All I know, AJ, is that Dr. Atkins says carbohydrates contribute to weight gain."

"It's not just people our age who are getting fatter," I responded. "Even my twelve-year-old son is putting on weight. Kids all over America weigh more than kids at the same age did thirty years ago. Something's going on here, but I don't think it's just carbs."

The waitress brought our bill, and as we walked to the parking lot, Gary stopped at the curb.

"Maybe you can figure it out, AJ. You're the chemical engineer. You know chemistry. What slows down the rate of a chemical reaction? Isn't that what metabolism is? The rate of a chemical reaction?"

I had to laugh. "Me? You're kidding! I know chemistry, but I'm certainly not a doctor. All these diet gurus seem to be doctors."

"Maybe that's why no one has found the answer," Gary said. "Maybe doctors don't have all the answers. Maybe what we need here is a different skill set. Besides, Pasteur wasn't a medical doctor, either."

Louis Pasteur was the nineteenth-century scientist who introduced the pasteurization of milk and developed vaccination as a method of preventing diseases.

"Pasteur wasn't a doctor? How did he come up with the idea of vaccinations?" I asked.

Gary went into the "teaching mode" I remembered so well from our college days.

"Pasteur observed people in an objective manner, noticing that some got sick while others—who had been exposed to weaker germs—seemed to build a type of immunity. He worked many hours in his laboratory and eventually came up with the theory that when weakened microbes were placed in an animal's body, the animal could actually build its own natural defenses to fight the microbe. As a result of his studies, humanity was able to save many lives from rabies, anthrax, and other diseases."

Gary looked closely at me. "You know people better than anyone I know. You have a knack for observing them and listening to them. I wish I could do it as well as you do. What's your secret, anyway?"

Smiling, I said, "Two things have really helped me. First, I've learned to be a good listener, and nobody ever complains of somebody listening too much. I have never heard a woman say, 'Oh, my husband listens too much,' or a man say, 'Oh, I can't stand my wife because every time I want to say something, she's ready and eager to listen to what I say.' So as a personal goal, I set out to become a master of the art of listening. I figured it wouldn't hurt my marriage to give my wife one less reason for complaining, you know?"

"I hear you."

"If you want to become an expert listener, just be as attentive to the other person as you can. Don't think about what you're going to say, just listen. The second thing that helped me to become a good listener is a quote from Rumi, a favorite Persian philosopher of mine from back in the thirteenth century. He wrote, 'Listen to what anyone says as though they were the last words of a father to his son. Listen with that much compassion, and you'll never feel jealousy or anger again.'" [1]

As we approached Gary's spotless new gas eater, I continued, "There's one more lesson I learned about the art of listening, Gary. Never prejudge a person by the way he looks."

Then I told him a story President Reagan had told me about

a king who had gone to the opening ceremony of a huge cathedral thirty years in the making.

All the people who had worked on the project were lined up to greet the king. First in line was the proud architect, who pointed out the inspiring design elements and uplifting contours he had given to the building. Next was the master builder, who showed the king the careful craftsmanship with which he had laid stone and marble, and the artistry with which he produced the awe-inspiring stained glass windows.

Last in line was an old man, a laborer, humbly dressed but also beaming with pride.

"And you, sir," the king asked, "what did you do on this magnificent project?"

"I was the lowliest part of a team that worked incredibly hard to build this great cathedral in which people from around the world can come to worship the Creator of all things beautiful," the old man said.

"You see, life is simply a matter of perspective. No matter who you are."

"My point exactly, AJ. And with your perspective as an engineer, a trained observer, you're just the guy to solve this dieting puzzle."

"And how would you suggest I do that?"

"Observe. Listen. Write down what you learn. If you find something in our eating habits today, compare it to years ago. See what has changed. Remember that study you did years ago, trying to determine why some of the thirty thousand people you talked to were successful while others were not? What did you learn?"

"I found five common traits of successful people," I answered. "They were (1) successful people have specific goals, (2) they have a plan, (3) they surround themselves with a support group, (4) they have can-do attitudes, and (5) they have plenty of energy."

"Well, if energy is supposed to come from food," Gary laughed, "it's sure not happening for me. I could take a nap!"

He eased himself into the car and rolled down his window.

"AJ, if you can find out why I'm not getting the energy I need out of my food, then you'd really have something. Is there a chemical reaction that's supposed to take place inside me that has stopped working? If so, what is it and why has it stopped?"

Watching Gary's car drive off, I was thoughtful. *Why was Gary not energized by his meal? Lots of people feel sluggish or sleepy after a meal, but why was that? Could that be related to gaining weight?*

On the way back to the office, I thought about how nice it would be if I did find a solution that dropped the twenty pounds or so I needed to lose and helped my son do the same. I stopped at a nearby convenience store and bought a soft drink out of the refrigerated display. The clerk, sipping a tall glass of water as she took my cash, was about twenty-five years old and about fifty pounds overweight.

Funny, I thought, *obesity is so commonplace it's become part of the landscape. I hardly notice it anymore.*

Grabbing a newspaper, I walked across the street to sit on a bench in a small park. A headline caught my eye: "Obesity is the second leading cause of preventable deaths." It was a story about a study reported in a major medical magazine, revealing that more than four hundred thousand people had died in this country during the year 2000 as a result of poor diet and lack of exercise. This pair ranked second only to smoking as a major cause of death in America.[2]

As I sat there in that park, I remember thinking I should have become a medical doctor. Had I done so, I might have been able to directly help more people. Instead, I pursued chemical engineering.

My mind wandered back some twenty years before, while in college. One of the prettiest girls in my class had asked for help in chemistry. "I can't figure out the difference between exothermic and endothermic reactions," she had said. "Can you help?"

Help a beautiful girl in a course filled with mostly male students? I quickly explained the difference in the two reactions. Endothermic reactions absorb heat as when you mix salt with an icy road. Exothermic reactions give out heat as when you mix acid and water. The girl gushed excitedly over the explanation then ran off.

Even twenty years later, I could vividly remember how my heart had pulsed with puppy love for that flighty young coed. A couple of weeks after we first spoke, I learned she was engaged to a football player named Jay, who just happens to be one of my oldest friends.

So much for helping people.

As I began to read more about the obesity problem, I discovered it was worse than I had imagined. More people were dying of obesity every year than had died during the entire Vietnam War, more people than had died at Hiroshima.

Helping people was ingrained in me. How could I not help them if it were in my power to do so? Then and there, I decided to fight the war against obesity. But where to begin? A quote from Abraham Lincoln came to mind: "The best way to destroy your enemy is to make him your friend."[3]

I decided to learn everything I could about the causes of obesity. I wasn't a medical doctor, but as Gary had pointed out, neither was Pasteur. I didn't have the knowledge that doctors have—and it was intimidating that so many diet books are written by MDs.

But how many of those diets are effective over time? So many people try fad diets like Atkins or South Beach, lose a few pounds, and quickly gain them all back. So much for diets written by doctors.

What, on the other hand, did I have to offer? A scientist with twenty-five years of experience in chemical engineering, I was known among colleagues and clients as a trained observer with a knack for looking at things outside the box. If medical doctors, dietitians, and nutritionists could not solve obesity after decades of trying, could an outside-the-box approach work any better? Were medical skills and clinical experience actually disadvantages rather than advantages? Were medical schools failing to give doctors the skill sets they needed to permanently solve obesity issues?

Perhaps the solution was not even related to nutrition. Maybe it was related to chemistry. The truth is, there are many similarities between the chemistry of the body and the chemistry found in the mechanical world. In many ways, the body is the perfect factory.

I began right then and there to put my observations into writing. What did I have for lunch? Fish and chips. What did Gary have? A hamburger with no bun. We both had drinks with the meal: iced tea for Gary and a glass of cola for me. But I sent that cola back because the glass had been two-thirds full of ice—a pet peeve of mine. Restaurants fill glasses with ice, so the amount of soda you receive is a fraction of what it should be. The menu reads "Glass of Pepsi, $1.25" not "1/3 glass of Pepsi plus 2/3 glass of ice, $1.25." When did restaurants start ripping off their customers with this game of ice robbery? How expensive can ice cubes be that restaurants charge so much for them?

I knew I would get nowhere if I allowed myself to wander off on things like the cost of ice cubes. *But what about the soda inside of the glass? Was soda the culprit? What had that obese clerk in the convenience store been drinking? Did it only look like water? Was it really soda?*

I walked back across the street to the convenience store and approached the clerk. "Excuse me," I started, "I'm doing a little research. Do you mind if I ask you if that's soda you're drinking there?"

"It's just water," the clerk responded, "and some ice, of course. The boss doesn't mind if I help myself to an occasional soda. But I never touch drinks with sugar in them. I'm trying to lose weight."

"It must be nice to work in a place where the drinks are free. Do you mind if I ask—for my research—whether your parents are heavy?"

"Well," the girl responded, "not until the last several years or so. But I've been heavy almost all my life. I've tried every diet I can find, but nothing seems to work. I get depressed, so I eat. If I could stop eating, I could drop this weight."

She took another sip. Leaving the store, I wrote down our conversation.

That evening I attended my son's Little League game. Watching the kids on the field, I counted the number of overweight boys. It came to about half of all the players in the game. Looking down the row at the other parents, the number was even higher: about three out of four.

Just then Randy, another of the parents, showed up, and I greeted him: "Randy, where have you been? The game's already started."

Randy winced apologetically. "Sorry, hope my kid didn't notice. But I got hung up in traffic. You know how slow the freeway traffic is this time of day."

"Did you stop for dinner?"

"You kidding? I just didn't have time. But I'm here and that's what is important."

Just then, Randy's son came to bat.

"Good eye!" Randy shouted as the boy stood immobile when the first nearly perfect home run pitch floated untouched into the catcher's mitt. "He's biding his time," Randy said, "just biding his time."

On the next pitch, the youngster clipped a corner of the ball and scrambled as it dribbled off toward third base. "Dig in, son, beat it out!" Randy was jumping up and down, and the entire bleacher section was on their feet in support. The boy crossed first just ahead of the ball, a two-bouncer from the frantic third baseman. The cheers were loud and long, carrying on that unspoken tradition of Little League parents that implied: if you cheer for everyone else's kid, everyone else has to cheer for yours.

"He's a natural, isn't he?" Randy said as the crowd settled back into their seats. "I do wish he weren't so heavy though. Not that I'm much better." He patted the roll of fat bulging over the top of his belt buckle. "I need to lose about thirty pounds. My doc says I've got high cholesterol. I know I need to exercise, but I don't have the time or energy anymore."

His wife, Sharon, had the same complaint: no energy. I was surprised to see that she was not overweight even though they were in the same family and presumably ate the same food.

During the next few months, I heard the same phrase over and over again. "No energy. No time to exercise." Each time, I noted the speaker's weight, plus his eating and drinking habits, and started filling up notebook pads with observations.

In public restaurants, at the mall—everywhere food is served —I tried to make sense out of what I was seeing. During this part of my research, 2,720 of the 2,823 adults I interviewed admitted that exercising was good for them. But only 132 people said they exercised regularly.

One day, while pouring my son a glass of milk, I noticed how cold the milk was. *Funny,* I thought, *when I was a kid, all the milk we drank was warm.*

What else was different about today and thirty or forty years ago? Everywhere I went this was the foremost question on my mind. At dinner with business associates, I questioned them about their eating habits. I asked each of them about how their diets and activity levels might have changed over the past few decades.

Observing other patrons at restaurants, I wrote down what each person was eating and drinking, noting whether they were overweight or not. When I could, I approached strangers and asked about their eating habits.

I became a regular at the local library, reading every book I could find on the subject of diets and dieting, spending hundreds of hours studying the experts and analyzing their studies and opinions. The earliest diet book I found was a 1918 bestseller entitled *Diet and Health with Key to the Calories,* by Dr. Lulu Hunt Peters. It was the first book to advocate calorie counting as a method of weight reduction.[4] Meantime, while doing this research, I still had to make a living. Out of the blue I received a call from Jay, my old college friend who had married the young coed who had caught my eye all those years ago. Jay was now an executive with a Texas firm and needed help with a new energy product they were developing.

Jay's associate, Brian, met me at the Dallas airport and suggested we have a quick lunch before meeting with Jay.

The restaurant was packed, and as we waited for a table, I studied the crowd. Life in Texas was apparently good—people were heavier than I remembered from the days when I lived there.

"It's not the same Texas you used to know," Brian said. "'God's Country' is in danger of becoming 'Fat Country.' We're all stressed out now. Jobs are going to China. Even this project you're helping us with, if it doesn't succeed, could result in five hundred people losing their jobs. Rumor is the plant may be shut down. It's getting scary."

"Don't worry, and don't be scared. Let me tell you a story that President Reagan told me."

A law was passed in California some years ago that required anyone working in public schools to be able to read and write. That especially affected one middle-aged school janitor who had never learned to read or write. When the principal discovered his inability, he fired him. With a little money he had saved, the man was able to buy some fruit to sell door-to-door. A couple of months later, he had enough money to buy a cart. Then two carts. Then he bought a small store, and after that, several more stores. It wasn't long before he was the richest man in town. One day he went to his bank to take out a million-dollar loan for yet another expansion.

The banker was delighted to help him. "Just fill out and sign this application," he said, "and we'll get things rolling."

"Sorry, but I can't."

"What do you mean? The money is ready for you, but you have to fill out this form. Just a formality, really."

"You don't understand, sir. I cannot read or write."

The banker was amazed. "A man with your wealth and business savvy, but you can't read or write? Preposterous!"

"Exactly."

"Can you imagine," the banker asked, "where you'd be if you had learned to read and write as a child?"

"Of course. I'd still be a janitor in a school in Los Angeles."

"So don't worry or be scared," I reassured Brian. "Trust God, have faith, and take risks. Now, what time are we due at the plant?"

Back at the company, we got down to business.

"We produce energy from waste materials we've collected," Jay said, "mostly old tires. We start with tires, plus a few plastic bottles and other garbage. We separate out the metals, and then we burn the nonmetals. The heat that generates creates mechanical energy, and we convert that into electricity."

(If you pay close attention to the details, you may find some clues to what's making America fat.)

"After the metals are separated out," Jay continued, "the nonmetals go into an open tank and then into a closed reactor. Acid and water are then added automatically to cause an exothermic reaction."

Exothermic, you remember, is the chemical reaction that releases energy in the form of heat, light, or sound. In this case, it's heat.

When the acid and water are in optimal amounts and oxygen is added at just the right time, the waste materials burn more efficiently, produce more heat, and ultimately produce more electrical energy. The problem in Jay's plant was that the end results were not sufficient to justify the costs.

It was important then to monitor the temperature levels in order to achieve optimum energy production. Determine the mix of ingredients that produces the most heat, I told Jay, and then monitor it closely to keep it at an optimal level.

Then it struck me how similar this was to the way our bodies produce energy from food. Were there some clues here?

Just after this meeting in Texas, I received a call from a European company whose operations were also losing money because in their manufacturing process, the reaction of dissolving photo resist—a photosensitive material used in manufacturing silicon chips in the semiconductor industry—was not taking place completely.

Hopping a plane to England, I soon found myself conducting tests at the ailing plant. Once again, I discovered that maintaining optimum temperatures was key in making the exothermic reaction take place completely. Yet company after company tended to overlook that fact and encountered productivity problems when they did.

Back home I continued to observe people for clues to the causes of weight gain. One Saturday I went to Costco on a shopping trip. Circling around for a parking spot closest to the door, it seemed as if everyone wanted the spots close to the entrance. I then noticed one car that parked at the very end of the lot. Trained to focus in on aberrations from the norm, I made a beeline to the spot right beside him. The driver was not young or athletic but was a middle-aged Asian man who appeared to be in good shape.

"Excuse me," I said, catching the man's attention. "I noticed you parking at the end of the lot while everyone else is waiting for a closer space. Would you mind if I ask you why you chose to park way out here?"

Startled, the man answered, "Why no, I always park in the first parking spot I come across, near or far. Is there a problem?"

"No, not at all. It's probably a good thing."

"You bet it is," the man replied. "If everybody did this, parking where they might have to walk a small distance, we'd save 2.5 millions of gallons of gasoline a day. Look at those cars over there circling around for a spot near the entrance. And look at the exercise opportunities those people are missing."

"I can't argue with that. Why don't people walk more? We could reduce pollution, save money, save gasoline, and be healthier. But people say they don't have the energy they used to."

"They need to eat more like Asians." The man laughed. "More rice, more bread. That's where people will find the energy they need. Energy for cars is limited; oil reserves will run out some day. But the energy that drives our bodies—carbohydrates—is unlimited."

With that, he briskly walked away.

My quest continued. One day in Phoenix, a waiter took my lunch order.

"Something to drink, sir?"

"No thanks."

"Nothing?"

"No, nothing. Thanks."

The waiter brought ice water anyway.

When did we start drinking so much ice water? I wondered. And what about cold foods like salads? Or all those other foods that cause an endothermic [absorbing heat] *rather than exothermic* [emitting heat] *reaction? Salty foods and sugar, for example, are all endothermic, especially when mixed with ice. They're absorbing the heat rather than emitting it. What can that mean?*

I also noted how often Americans eat cold foods before hot foods. In restaurants, waiters routinely serve cold drinks first, whether a cold soda, iced tea, or ice water. More often than not, the first food placed on the table is a cold salad.

What happens inside the human body when something cold is introduced to the stomach? Does it matter? Was I spinning my wheels with this line of questioning? The frustration began to wear on me.

Watching television one Sunday morning, I was channel surfing when I happened across a dynamic Houston, Texas, preacher, Pastor Joel Osteen of Lakewood Church, calmly but confidently addressing his congregation: "Good things flow from adversity."

A couple of channels later and another minister—Dr. Creflo Dollar—was saying, "Wisdom is how you use your knowledge."

Those two messages stayed in my mind. I felt as if the two preachers were speaking directly to me. It was true: the project was beginning to wear down on me. Thousands of observations and pads full of notes, yet I had not yet found the answer. I was spending so much time trying to find a solution to the weight-gain problem that even my business was threatened.

Walking out onto the patio, I sank dejectedly into a padded chair.

"I'm so tired, Lord," I prayed, lowering my face into my hands. "Thank you for getting me involved in this project, but I don't know if I can complete it. I don't know what to do. Lord, how can I continue?"

Opening my eyes, a small movement caught my eye. Looking down, I saw a caterpillar inching slowly along the ground toward the bushes. How slow, yet how determined and focused this tiny creature was. Over my shoulder, more motion caught my eye. It was a delicate little hummingbird darting quickly from flower to flower. How amazing these little creatures are, how steady they are as they fly in place. What keeps them going?

Suddenly, a shaft of soft and shimmering colors pierced down through a patch of sunlight through the tree branch overhead. Looking up, I saw the most beautiful rainbow I had ever seen.

It was as if God was sending me a soft touch on the shoulder, a priceless gift of encouragement: Be persistent. Keep working. Remain focused. And the most beautiful results will be opened to you.

Reinvigorated, I carried on.

Soon afterward, my travels again took me to London. Eating dinner in a quaint little restaurant a block or so from my hotel, I began to observe the people around me.

The first thing that struck me was that there were fewer overweight or obese people than I was accustomed to seeing back in the States. Were the English thinner than Americans? I watched as the patrons sat down at nearby tables, peacefully sipping hot tea while waiting for their food. Few if any had a cold salad. The main entrées were all hot foods and served in much smaller portions than what I had witnessed back home.

In a Paris restaurant a couple of days later, I noted similar results. The locals seemed to be much slimmer than my fellow citizens back home. Glancing over the menu, I selected the house specialty: hot soup of the day, an appetizer followed by salad, the main entrée, and dessert—topped off with a glass of red wine. I also noticed that many of the diners seemed to be electing for a nice walk up and down the boulevard after dinner rather than rushing home to watch television. *Now this is truly relaxing,* I thought as I sipped the hot soup.

As with most French restaurants, if you wanted water, you had to ask for it. No one automatically served ice water. Not long after I began to eat, I heard a commotion at a table a few feet away. An angry American businessman was indignantly demanding ice water. "What kind of place is this," the portly, red-faced man was demanding, "where you can't even get ice water with your meal? For crying out loud, aren't you people civilized?"

For the rest of his meal, the American grumbled loudly to all who could hear about the poor service. "The food's not that great either," the man sputtered as he quickly shoveled forkfuls of food into his mouth. "Look at these stingy little portion sizes! You guys ever hear of man-sized portions?" He washed it all down with large gulps of the water he had so loudly demanded. Eyes darting around the room, he challenged anyone to give him further reason for battle.

The waiters seemed to steer clear of the troublesome visitor. I heard one say, "No wonder nobody likes these Americans! All they care about is their silly ice water. Why can't they slow down and relax?"

What is it, I wondered, *that other countries know about dieting that Americans do not?* They are relatively trim; we are increasingly fat. Asians are trim, too, I remembered, thinking back to my trips to Japan. What is so different about diets in those countries versus our own? And when foreigners immigrate to the U.S., why do so many of them seem to gain weight?

Is it the portion sizes we Americans have come to expect in our restaurants and in our homes? Is that how we are destroying ourselves? Is there some kind of international conspiracy to make our nation ineffective by making us overweight?

I pictured a lanky Osama Bin Laden sponsoring television campaigns encouraging Americans to "Super-size it! Super-size it! Eat your way to oblivion, American jackals!"

That was ridiculous, of course.

On the flight home, I sat between two ladies. The conversation turned to dieting and the possible causes behind America's out-of-control waistlines. One lady ordered a glass of ice water (*Here we go again*, I thought), and the other lady ordered orange juice and ice. When the orange juice was gone, she chewed on the ice as they spoke. Both ladies were veterans of the diet wars. Both had strong opinions about carbohydrates versus proteins. If someone could just find a way to lose weight without making you give up your favorite foods, both agreed, then you'd really have something.

For almost five years, these were the types of comments and experiences I gathered from countless conversations and observations. We needed a solution. But what could it possibly be?

I began to dig even deeper into the problem. I took all the clues and then applied what I had learned to biochemistry—the study of chemical substances and vital processes as they occur in living organisms. I took the information I had gathered over those years and applied it to the chemical processes that take place within the body, especially within the digestive tract.

I read everything I could find on the digestive process. What happens chemically when food is ingested into the body? What chemical process has to take place for proper digestion? What prevents food from being fully digested, and when the digestion is less than 100 percent, how does that impact the body?

I had long discussions with biochemical engineers. Adapting what I knew from my experience in chemical engineering, I created numerous theses about what biochemical reasons might be behind American weight problems today versus forty years ago.

Undeniably, we are exercising less. Why is that? Is it television—or something more subtle? What is robbing us of the energy we need to exercise?

We are also eating much larger portions than we did forty years ago. Why is that? Why don't we feel full after a few minutes and stop eating? Are we deriving less energy from the food we eat?

What has happened to us over the decades that led to today's problems?

"OK, AJ," I said, edging forward on my seat, "so what's the answer? You discovered the answer, you said. What did you learn about the secret to losing weight?"

"It's more simple than anyone could imagine, Bill," AJ said, taking a sip from his drink. "Incredibly simple. But it's the most logical thing in the world when you hear the reason why."

"What is it?"

"Bill, the reason Americans are gaining so much weight, the secret to successfully losing weight and maintaining your goal weight for the rest of your life . . ."

"Yes?"

"Without starving yourself or going hungry . . ."

"Yeah?"

"Without giving up any major food group or your favorite foods . . ."

"Right . . ."

"Including your favorite sweets. The poison that is sapping our lost energy . . ."

"Come on, AJ!"

He smiled. Then he picked up something from the table and laid it flat in his hand.

"It's right here, Bill. This is the poison."

Wide-eyed, I stared down at the small object nestled in his palm.

"Who could have guessed?" he said.

3: THE DISCOVERY

ce?" I stared at the ice cube in his hand. "Ice is the poison? Ice is making us fat?"

"Not just ice," AJ said, slipping the dripping cube from one hand to the other, "but what ice does to your metabolism. Let me be clear: we're talking about ice or icy drinks consumed along with food. An ice drink taken without food does not constitute nearly the same problem."

"So a glass of iced cola—without food—on a hot day is OK?"

"Yes, Bill. Even though there may be sugar in that drink, it's the ice that is the problem. Not the sugar. Of course, you've got to watch the calories from the sugar. You have to drink in moderation."

AJ leaned forward intently, his hand still dripping from the melting ice.

"You and I are getting fat because, when we drink icy cold beverages or eat icy cold foods, we disrupt our bodies' digestive process and slow down metabolism, which is how food turns into energy. Without energy, we become sedentary. We sit rather than walk. We walk rather than run—and what little walking we do is never as far as it was when we were younger. We take cars where we used to walk. As a result of the vicious cycle this behavior sets up, millions of Americans are adding weight. And for the vast majority of those of us who are overweight or obese, the problem begins right here, with this tiny ice cube."

I glanced around at the tables near me. With more than a little skepticism, I found myself wondering, *Was this possible? Is ice wrecking havoc with our diets? Is ice the poison that's killing Americans?*

Sure enough, virtually every diner had a frosty glass of iced tea, ice water, or soda next to his plate. One man gulped down half a glass of ice water even before his meal arrived.

I thought back to before I began AJ's seven-day diet. Most of my meals included some kind of cold drink such as cold soda, iced tea, or just plain water with ice cubes from the refrigerator. Sometimes I even chewed ice.

Slowly I pushed my glass back from my plate. "I've had ice with my drinks for years."

"Exactly. You almost cannot order a beverage these days—including water—without it being served in a glass brimming with ice. I bet you didn't have much ice as a skinny kid in Wisconsin, did you?"

"No. Except maybe with Kool-Aid or lemonade. Mom rarely bought canned soda back then. It was a special treat when she did."

"I'll also bet your mom didn't serve cold salads on frozen plates, did she?"

"No. We usually had hot soup before the main course. Dad used to say life was good if you were getting three warm meals a day."

"And what about at school? What beverage did you have with lunch?"

"Sometimes milk but usually just water."

"Guess what they serve in school lunchrooms these days."

"Cold drinks?"

"Exactly. Cafeterias are lined with machine after machine dispensing ice-cold cans of sugar-enriched, calorie-packed sodas and juice. Kids chug those drinks down with their food, all the time talking excitedly to one another, getting all animated, never experiencing any kind of internal calm whatsoever. And when the kids come home, they grab a cold soda out of the fridge and flop down in front of their computers to play computer games for five hours. Is it any wonder kids are packing on pounds faster than ever before in history?"

I thought about one of the first times I had an ice-filled soda—aside from the occasional lemonade served by my mother. It was back in my high school days, back in the sixties. Drive-in restaurants were highly popular, and it was a big deal to drive up with a car full of guys, ogle the carhops, and fork over a buck-ninety-five for a burger, fries, and soft drink. We squeezed as many as five or six guys into those old cars. It helped that no one was overweight or obese.

"You think our weight problems started back in the fifties and sixties," I asked, "when fast-food restaurants first became popular?"

"Fast food was one factor. The entrées are typically filled with all kinds of empty calories and unhealthy ingredients. But other contributing factors included meals designed to be eaten on the run, washed down by tall, sugar-filled sodas brimming with ice cubes," AJ said, settling back in his chair.

"So to lose weight, all I have to do is stop drinking iced drinks?"

"Not quite, but that would be a start. Ice is, well, only the tip of the iceberg. The core problem is that when we eat, we're cooling down our body at a time when it absolutely must be warm in order for the digestive process to work efficiently. If you want to lose weight, you need a diet that includes lots of warm foods and warm drinks. It's what I call the 'Hot Diet.'"

I still didn't get it. "What does heat have to do with the way I digest my food? And what's this Hot Diet anyway?"

"One question at a time. First, let me tell you how heat helps break down food and converts it to energy."

— BEFORE FOOD IS EATEN, TINY BONDS THAT GIVE THE FOOD shape and substance hold it together. Once ingested, these bonds are gradually broken down, starting with saliva in the mouth and continuing with chemicals in the stomach. Once broken down, the food is then converted into energy that drives the body.

The walls of the stomach contain a group of cells called the *parietal* cells. Their job is to secrete the hydrochloric acid that digests the food. Ice, cold fluids, and cold foods can have a numbing effect on these cells, preventing them from working efficiently.

Many years ago ice was used to treat stomach ulcers. To ease the pain, doctors would recommend eating lots of ice. It worked like a natural anesthesia. When you pour your icy sodas into your stomach, is it any wonder that the parietal cells are shocked by the low temperatures and produce hydrochloric acid at a much slower rate than nature intended?

If the parietal cells are not producing hydrochloric acid—even temporarily—ingested food cannot be digested efficiently. The meat or vegetables you eat will sit in your stomach anywhere from a few minutes to a few hours longer than they would if you had not consumed the ice. The problem with this is that your body has to expend energy rewarming the stomach to its normal body temperature—using energy you normally would use to engage in after-meal exercise or activities.

So think about what happens: You drink the cold fluids—shutting down or restricting the parietal cells. The body has to waste energy bringing internal temperatures back to normal. So after dinner you don't have the energy you need to move about—exercise, walk around the block, and so forth—to work off calories from the meal. During the course of several years, this pattern results in a gradual weight gain and, because you don't have the energy to exercise, a corresponding loss in calorie-consuming muscle mass.

The weight gain happens gradually at first. Most of us don't even notice it. But over the years, a pound or two of extra weight adds up to thirty or forty pounds before you know it.

Consuming ice starts a chain reaction that makes your digestive system less efficient, steals your energy, and forces you to alter your previous activity patterns. Ever so gradually, you become less active. More and more calories turn to fat instead of energy. Your muscles, which are incredible twenty-four-hour-a-day fat burners, become less massive. And one day you wake up and realize you're fat.

Remember the story about my wife bringing me the glass of iced tea by the pool? That's the day it hit me like lightning. Looking at the ice cube floating in the tea, I suddenly realized the answer. Gaining weight isn't just about the foods we eat— food is only part of the problem. Gaining weight is not solely about the amount of sugar or salt we consume, or about good carbs versus bad carbs. Gaining weight is about the biochemical problems we create when we obstruct the naturally efficient conversion of food to energy. And that's exactly what ice does.

In observations of more than 104,700 people, including those who were visibly overweight and those who were not, I recorded what each person was drinking or eating just before, during, and after their meals.

What I found was startling:

Weight Class	Total	Drank Ice Water/Beverage*	Percent
Regular weight	26,493	7,322	27.6%
Overweight/obese	78,207	73,155	93.5%

*Some diners had nothing to drink.

An astonishing 93.5 percent of people who were visibly overweight or obese were drinking ice water or ice-filled beverages, versus only 27.6 percent of people who appeared to be of regular weight levels. Ten times as many visibly overweight diners drank cold beverages than people who were not overweight.

As I reviewed this and other data, I was struck by the simplicity of the answer. The link between weight gain and cold beverages—or cold foods—was as obvious as the arrow in the FedEx logo. How could so many diet "experts" have missed the mark so widely? Was it because so few of the diet gurus are certified nutritionists or dietitians—or was it also because the culprit is not related to food but to chemistry?

For years now, diet books have sent people on wild goose chases. How many times have you heard that you should or should not eat meat or grains or sugar or a hundred other things? Who knows what to believe anymore? Our ancestors did just fine when they ate balanced meals. Fad diets fail for one very important reason: they think food is the problem, but when taken in proper portions, it really isn't.

With the Hot Diet, you can actually fine-tune the digestive process so that your metabolism is boosted to its highest levels of efficiency. You can eat virtually any food you want, without starving yourself, without suffering even the slightest as the pounds melt away. But calories do matter. They always have and always will. If you eat more calories than your body needs, you will add weight. Excess calories inevitably end up stored in your body as fat. But when you follow the Hot Diet and get your digestive process working the way nature intended, you'll be eating the healthiest, most natural diet of your life, with more energy than you ever imagined possible, and you'll be as trim as you want to be.

What about the science behind this theory? Let me describe what happens when we ingest food. First let's revisit those two types of chemical reactions: exothermic and endothermic. An *exothermic* reaction gives off heat. For example, burning wood is a chemical process that produces heat, as does mixing vinegar and baking soda. An *endóthermic* reaction absorbs heat. A boiling egg, for example, absorbs heat and becomes hard.

The relationship between food, heat, and energy has long been established. In 1842, a German physician and physicist named Julius von Mayer observed that people in different climates needed different amounts of food to maintain their body temperatures. In hotter climates, people needed less food; in colder climates, they needed more. This helped establish the theory—later proven—that there is a direct relationship between the consumption of food and the generation of heat. Not well presented at the time, Mayer's theory was at first discounted by the scientific community but later supported by other studies.

A year or so after Mayer released his theory, James Prescott Joule published a work describing the interchangeable nature of motion and heat, demonstrating that any specific type of work would always generate the same amount of heat. Food, heat, and exercise, therefore, were intricately linked from that day forward.

When we eat, food is transformed into heat (or energy). When we move about, we use up that energy.

In human digestion, all chemical reactions are exothermic—

they generate or release heat. It is through the generation of heat that our bodies create the energy that enables us to move, walk, or otherwise change positions. If the exothermic reaction does not take place completely or efficiently, less energy is produced and it is more difficult to move about.

Think of a log in a fireplace. If it's not positioned properly, the log can't get the oxygen it needs to burn. It doesn't put out nearly as much heat—energy—as it could if the oxygen were available in optimum quantities. The body's exothermic process is the same way. By ingesting cold fluids or foods, you prevent the body from dispensing the chemicals necessary for digestion. Instead of energy from the food becoming available for physical activities, a critical portion of it is used to rewarm the body. Lacking energy, you plop down in the easy chair after a big meal instead of walking, running, working, or playing.

Again, this takes place over months or years. A single ice water drink with food, for example, might have only a negligible effect. The problem comes when we habitually consume icy fluids with food over a long period of time. The average person drinks about twenty thousand gallons of cold water and other liquids in his or her lifetime, according to my calculations. Can you imagine the energy it takes to warm up 20,000 gallons of water to 98.6 degrees? All that energy is no longer available for doing your housework, mowing the lawn, chasing after the kids, playing golf—you name it. It's like slowly letting the air out of a tire. Sooner or later, the car is going to have a flat, and movement will become very difficult.

So how do we turn all of this around? How do we get our bodies operating at peak performance again? First, let's look at how heat works on the mechanical side. As a chemical engineer, I appreciate the role of heat in achieving an optimal chemical reaction. Look at the simple process of building a really good campfire. There are five principles of successful campfire building:

LOG BURNING PRINCIPLE #1:

Use the best components you can find. If the wood is damp, it's a poor candidate for a fire. Certain types of wood ignite more easily, and certain combinations of wood (such as soft wood intermingled with hard wood) burn hotter and produce more heat.

LOG BURNING PRINCIPLE #2:

Introduce the wood at an optimal rate. If you add logs to the fire too quickly, it may go out. Add logs too slowly and the result is the same. But if you add logs at just the right pace, you will achieve a better flame and generate more heat.

LOG BURNING PRINCIPLE #3:

Keep pressure at an optimum level. Different pressure levels yield different results. For example, it's harder to build a fire at higher elevations. When pressure is changed, the rate of chemical reaction also changes.

LOG BURNING PRINCIPLE #4:

Stir the logs for a better burn. When you agitate the position of logs in the fireplace, they get more oxygen and burn faster. For a hotter fire, stoke it frequently.

LOG BURNING PRINCIPLE #5:

Keep the fire burning hot. The higher the heat, the more thoroughly the fire consumes the logs. Every chemical reaction has an optimum temperature, but as a general rule, the rate of reaction doubles for every ten-degree (centigrade) rise in temperature. A strong fire burns the logs completely while a weak fire leaves them half burned and smoldering.

That's the physical world. Now what about the biophysical world—the natural processes that take place within our bodies? How might those five principles of building a log fire apply to the digestive process? I found myself studying everything I could on the digestive process. I spent dozens of hours in libraries reading medical journals. I interviewed biochemists and physicians. Soon I began to understand and appreciate just what happens when we eat and digest food.

Digestion begins in the mouth. First your teeth change the shape and consistency of the food and reduce it in size. The longer you chew the food and grind it down, the easier it is to dissolve in your stomach. Your saliva moistens the food and converts it to a softer, more liquid state.

The chewed food then goes down through a hollow tube called the esophagus directly into the stomach. This is where digestion begins in earnest. As soon as food arrives in the stomach, hydrochloric acid (HCl) is released by the parietal cells to start breaking down the proteins. The muscles in the stomach, sensing there is something to work on, begin to crunch the food.

Eventually the food is transformed into a liquid form called *chyme.* It contains acid and gets neutralized with sodium bicarbonate, which is the same as baking soda. Next the digestive process is completed by pancreatic juice, bile, and intestinal juice. Fats and carbohydrates are broken down into smaller units. Then everything moves through a small ring called the pyloric sphincter directly into the small intestine, which is only an inch or so in diameter but more than twenty feet long. Its function is to allow only liquid to pass.

All of these chemical reactions require both water and oxygen to break down and release the energy in the food. The digested food enters the blood from the small intestine and liver and dissolves in plasma, which is the liquid part of blood. It is the blood that carries food and oxygen to cells throughout the body. Blood also carries carbon dioxide (CO_2) waste.

The large intestine stores waste and is much shorter than the small intestine, but it is more than two times as wide. Very little chemical reaction takes place in the large intestine. This process is basically the same in any living organism. Energy must be generated from chemical compounds in the food, and chemical reactions must take place before the energy can be released.

That's a somewhat simplified description of how food is turned into energy. Human chemistry is more complicated than laboratory chemistry. But the physical and chemical properties of the compounds are exactly the same as in the lab. That's why we need to know a lot more about organic chemistry, thermodynamics, and biology.

Unfortunately, medical doctors rarely if ever study thermodynamics, which covers the relationship between heat and other energy forms. Medical schools need to establish a new course of study called "bio-thermodynamics." This program would help young doctors understand the critical importance of chemical reactions within the digestive process and their ultimate impact upon body weight.

Can you imagine how much better doctors would be at treating overweight patients if they truly understood what happens to ingested food in the body? We wouldn't have any more wild goose chases over diets that pit proteins against carbohydrates. We wouldn't have people dieting on cabbages, or fasting and skipping meals, as their weight bounces up and down like a yo-yo.

Did you know that many medical doctors receive only twenty-five hours of training in nutrition? That's hardly enough to understand these sometimes complex relationships. If you rely on your doctor for nutritional advice, you have to wonder how knowledgeable he is. Some doctors are undoubtedly extremely well versed in nutrition—but most are not. Personally, I work with a highly qualified nutritionist, and I absolutely marvel at the depth of her knowledge in this area. She's spent a lifetime in study and practice. You can't compare twenty-five hours of training to that.

Recently, major organizations such as the American Society for Clinical Nutrition and the American Medical Student Association have called for more emphasis on nutrition education for medical students. Despite this, U.S. medical schools (with some notable exceptions) often fall short of the recommended twenty-five hours. Cynics might see the ubiquitous hand of pharmaceutical companies in this shortfall. Would drug companies lose big-time if physicians were recommending better eating habits and increased physical activity rather than prescribing drugs? You bet they would. Billions of dollars could be at stake if drugs were no longer the recommended solution for obesity and the many diseases that result from it.

One day medical schools will wake up and start offering studies like bio-thermodynamics in their course lists. The drug companies may hate it, but patients will benefit enormously.

Water plays a vital role in human chemistry. All plants and animals, including humans, need water to stay alive. It is used in virtually every step of digestion, from the first time a morsel of food enters our mouths to the time it leaves our bodies as waste. Water helps make all the necessary chemical reactions happen.

We need between seven and ten glasses of water every day, depending upon our weight. The average American should be drinking eight glasses, though most of us fall far short of that. Studies have shown that drinking enough water daily can decrease the risk of colon cancer by almost 50 percent. The same is true for bladder cancer and breast cancer (80 percent reduction in risk).[1]

But not just any water will do.

Warm water actually works better than cold water in starting the reaction that loosens bonds in the food and releases its energy. This process is called the *energy of activation*. It reinforces the reason the Hot Diet works so well in making our digestive process more efficient than ever.

Remember those five principles of fire burning? Let's compare log burning with food conversion.

Converting Wood to Heat	Converting Food to Energy
1. Use the best components you can find.	1. Eat a healthy, well-balanced diet.
2. Introduce components at an optimal rate.	2. Eat in moderation, slowly and calmly.
3. Keep pressure at an optimum level.	3. Minimize stress in your life.
4. Stir the logs for a better burn.	4. Exercise.
5. Keep the fire burning hot.	5. Avoid ice. Turn on the Hot Diet.

Natural laws are the same, both in nature and in the body, so it's no surprise that there are similarities in generating heat in a campfire and heating up your digestive process. As you will soon discover, this table forms the basis for the Hot Diet.

Before we get to that, however, we need to do some housecleaning. Sixty-eight percent of Americans have problems with their digestive tracts at one time or another, so it is critical to keep them clean and efficient. Theoretically, your intestines should be cleared before the next meal in order to more easily process the new food. In a perfect world, if you have three meals a day, that would mean three clean-outs.

The easiest way to clear your digestive tract is to drink warm water before, during, and after each meal.

You'll notice that throughout the Hot Diet, warmer fluids are always suggested instead of colder fluids. Part of the reason is that warm water (containing heat) promotes beneficial chemical processes while cold water does not.

Another problem is that the colder the water the more fat cells it attracts. The tendency to develop fat cells in response to cold temperatures is seen throughout nature. Just look at seals, whales, polar bears, and other mammals living in very cold locations. As part of their natural protection, they develop thick layers of fat. But since that fat is located just under the skin, acting as both insulation against heat loss and as an energy reserve, it's not damaging to the animal.

For most people, however, excess fat around the stomach and internal organs is a serious matter. This kind of fat poses a distinct danger because it makes the heart work harder and contributes to clogged arteries.

The stomach empties in about three to five hours after food is consumed, so warm beverages consumed during this time can be most beneficial. Mid-morning and mid-afternoon breaks are ideal for sipping hot tea or drinking very warm water, perhaps with a lemon wedge to give it some flavor. In other countries, this has been a tradition for centuries. Countries that take breaks for things like drinking tea do not have weight problems nearly as serious as ours.

For example, the English take their afternoon tea seriously. It was reported that when the English were about to do battle with the Spanish, back when Henry the Eighth was king, they paused for hot tea. When asked why, they responded, "Because it's not just civilized, but necessary." After tea they proceeded to destroy the Spanish.

The Chinese and Europeans in general prefer hot tea over iced tea. But even that is changing. Beverage industry experts report that the amount of iced tea served is starting to increase dramatically.[2]

In France, a country that never previously had a problem

with obesity, 11.3 percent of the French are now obese and nearly 40 percent are overweight.[3] I thought at one time that they were about five to seven years behind us in obesity levels, but they seem to be catching up fast. The belief that something in the French lifestyle protects them against obesity, heart disease, and diabetes is now fading into history. And whoever suggested that the French don't get fat may have spoken too soon. French women do get fat, and so do French men.

Causes of the weight change in France as cited by experts include the lure of fast food and prepared foods—the ubiquity of unhealthy snacks and sedentary lives. Somewhat telling, perhaps, is the success of McDonald's in France. Sales are booming. Some 1.2 million French—2 percent of the population—now eat at McDonald's every day.[4]

In England, similar stories are now hitting the media. Half of the men and a third of the women in England are overweight. And an additional 21 percent of men and 23 percent of women are categorized as obese.[5]

The epidemic may not yet be as obvious in France or England, but as poor eating habits, lack of exercise, and ice addiction continue to increase, that, too, will change.

HOT DIET PRINCIPLES

The diet revolves around five principles:

HOT DIET PRINCIPLE #1: EAT A BALANCED DIET.

Eat well. Do not neglect any major food group, and do not favor one food group over another. Forget high protein versus low carbs. Juggling proteins and carbs is far too dangerous, with too many long-term unknowns. Base your choice of foods on a highly balanced mix of good nutrition, variety, and moderation.

I recommend going back to the kind of foods we ate forty or fifty years ago, before we were caught up in fad diets. The food pyramid created by the U.S. Department of Agriculture is a good starting place. Eat lots of fruits, vegetables, beans, and whole grains. But to get your body working at peak efficiency, work in plenty of foods designed to speed up metabolism. In my research, I sought out some of the best dietitians in the country to develop an attractive, well-balanced menu that a person could confidently follow the rest of his or her life.*

The Hot Diet is built around keeping your body naturally warm. Never cool it down during food ingestion. Always eat foods that complement your body's need for warmth and for efficient metabolism.

Take Bill as an example. In his very first week, he lost weight and experienced a noticeable surge in energy. His seven-day diet included no icy drinks, only tea or hot chocolate with meals, and he did not miss the ice even for a minute.

This diet gets even better in weeks to come as you get past that phase where you want to drop weight and need only to maintain. You can eat almost anything—within reason, of course

One of my most important rules: *never ever skip breakfast.*

My research showed again and again that breakfast must be the biggest meal of the day. But rather than cereal soaking in cold milk, start with hot cereal, eggs, bacon (in limited

---

*A twenty-eight–day starter diet along with recommended daily menus plus Hot Diet recipes are included later in this book.

quantities), sausages, and so forth. Hot foods are more likely to stay with you for several hours. Always include a warm drink although juices are fine.

Lunch should be your second largest meal of the day, with about half to two-thirds the portion sizes of breakfast. Again, hot foods are better than cold foods, preferably washed down with a warm drink. Even though you're eating smaller amounts, warm drinks increase your sense of satisfaction with what you've had. You'll walk away from the table with a pleasant, completely content feeling that will remain with you throughout much of the afternoon.

Make dinner your lightest meal of the day. For best results, eat more carbohydrates than protein because you want a slow burn, and you're usually less active in the evening or during the night.

If you feel it necessary to eat more than three meals a day, do so. For example, add a small meal in mid to late afternoon. It can be a snack such as fruit or a handful of nuts, or perhaps a small serving of vegetables. As always, wash it down with hot tea, hot chocolate, or warm water.

Long ago, a Turkish lady gave me a good rule to follow: "Eat breakfast with family, lunch with friends, and dinner with enemies." So I try to eat breakfast with family, lunch with friends and friendly business associates, and save dinner for any tough negotiating I may have to do or any other less-than-friendly environment so I don't eat too much.

HOT DIET PRINCIPLE #2: EAT IN MODERATION.

Take your time. Keep portions small. Most of us eat far more food than we need. Eat slowly. As in the log fire example where introducing materials too fast could snuff the flame, always regulate the speed with which you eat. Eat at a moderate speed, slowly and calmly, chewing the food thoroughly. I recommend fifteen chews per morsel, even if you're eating at a fast-food restaurant.

Fast food doesn't mean you have to eat fast.

By taking your time, you not only let saliva do its part in moistening the food, but you also make it easier on your stomach. The nerves in the mouth signal the brain that food is being processed, which orders the acid in the stomach so it can react immediately when the food arrives. It is also important to remember that it takes twenty minutes for the brain to signal your body that you are full. When you eat too fast, you don't get the signal in time to quit when you should. Additionally, when you eat foods slowly you give them a chance to get closer to body temperature before they actually enter the stomach.

HOT DIET PRINCIPLE #3: MINIMIZE STRESS IN YOUR LIFE.

America is a particularly stressful society, far more so than it was thirty or forty years ago. You can see it in increased family tensions. (We seem to be fighting more today than we did decades ago. Do we have more to fight about?) You can see it in the changing eating habits of families where different members are missing from the table—at soccer practice, working late, stuck in traffic. If you think this does not apply to your own family, try to remember the last time your meal was a pleasant, relaxing occasion.

When you're under pressure, your digestive system cannot

work at maximum efficiency. The body has to work harder to raise the temperature of ingested foods and fluids. If you're truly committed to controlling your weight, you have to commit to eliminating stress as much as possible, but especially at mealtime.

When you eat, create an atmosphere of serenity, happiness, love, and joy. The best environment for a meal is a relaxed one, without anger, hate, fear, anxiety, or hurry. The worst possible way to begin a family meal could well be to pose the question: "Sooo . . . how was your day?" It's difficult to be calm when you remind yourself of the guy who cut you off on the freeway or the neighbor whose dog keeps soiling your showcase lawn.

Of the more than 104,000 people I observed while they were eating, more than 99,000 ate in a hurried fashion or engaged in animated conversations while they ate. Some even talked on their cell phone or watched TV. Only 5,213 appeared to be in a calm, peaceful state.

Stress can produce all kinds of negative effects within the body. It can build up fat in the abdominal area. It can cause stomach and intestinal pain, sleep disorders, and increased risk of heart disease. These are proven, indisputable facts with but one lesson for us all: *cut the stress or live with the fat.* Reduce the stress and you dramatically improve your chances of living a longer, happier life. As an added bonus, you may also lose some weight.

HOT DIET PRINCIPLE #4: EXERCISE.

You cannot get away from it: if you want to lose weight, you absolutely must exercise. The Hot Diet strongly supports exercise as a primary component of dieting success. Chemical reactions need movement or agitation to work efficiently, just as you need to stir the coals in a fire to keep it burning brightly. Agitation creates heat, which helps loosen the old bonds so the new bonds can be formed.

When you drop a lump of sugar into your cold water, what happens? It just sits there. But if you put the sugar into a glass of hot tea, it would melt.

Going back to your glass of cold water, if I stirred it with a spoon, the ice would melt in that case too. That's because motion generates heat inside your glass, and the heat melts the sugar lump. The faster you stir, the faster the sugar melts. The same thing happens inside the body when you exercise.

For certain chemical reactions in the human body to occur, therefore, there must be movement or physical exercise. For most of us, that means getting up, walking around, and occasionally lifting moderately heavy items.

An old proverb says, "From walking, something. From sitting, nothing."

There's a lot of truth in that. Why do we sit so much as a society? Many people say it's because they lack the energy to do anything else. So they relax for "just a little while," sipping on a cold drink and snacking while watching television. Two hours later, they are still there and even more tired.

But when you move your body, when you exercise, you stimulate chemical processes that produce even more energy. It's a beautiful system. Unfortunately, it's out of whack for most of us.

HOT DIET PRINCIPLE #5: AVOID ICE.

Eliminating ice is critical to the Hot Diet. It's like the keystone in an arch where balanced food selection, portion control, reduced stress, and exercise make up the lower portion of the arch, and ice avoidance supports both sides from the top.

Starting immediately, avoid cold beverages of all types when eating. Add a warm drink to every meal. After the meal, take your warm cup of tea or chocolate into the living room for a few minutes. Sit down and relax. Leave the TV off. Reflect on the great food you had. While you do, your body is working at maximum efficiency. Soon you will feel a surge of energy that you can use to take your daily walk, play with the kids, work around the yard, or do any number of things instead of just sitting there.

It is better to drink warm water or beverages before starting the meal, or in lieu of that, to drink nothing at all. Don't forget your eight glasses of water a day, but make sure the water, if you're eating food with it, is not ice cold.

Why do so many people drink ice-cold water or beverages before starting a meal? The temperature of everything you eat or drink should be the same as your body temperature or a little higher. I recommend 40 degrees Centigrade or 104 degrees Fahrenheit, which is just a bit higher than your body temperature. Why? Because energy always flows from a higher temperature to a lower one. If your drink is a little warmer than your body, that heat tends to flow to the body.

What do you do on a really hot day?

Make sure you drink lots of slightly cool fluids without any ice. If you still feel hot, go for a swim or take a cold shower rather than pouring cold water or beverages into your stomach. In a cold shower, for example, the body will produce heat inside and moderate your outside temperature more efficiently than a cold drink ever could. Producing this internal heat results in the melting of stored fat cells, and that's very beneficial when you're overweight.

Unfortunately, most of us do exactly the opposite. We cool our insides with ice-cold fluids and warm the outside with a hot bath or shower. Always use the body as your heat source, which requires it to use stored energy cells—fat. You will feel better, will have more energy, and could even increase the number of healthy, active years you spend on the planet.

Note how active people turn themselves into energy-burning machines. Many swimmers live longer than the rest of the population, and many swim well into their eighties or nineties. One active lady I ran in to during my travels was an avid swimmer—at one hundred and three years old.

Again, always cool the body from the outside, not the inside, and always keep hydrated.

It is also important to select foods that promote regularity. Make sure your diet includes a good amount of fiber so you can clean out your pipes. You can have salads on the Hot Diet, but I suggest you avoid very cold salads. Salads are great sources of fiber, so if you can, have your salad served at room temperature, or consider delaying it until after your main course as many Europeans do. And always wash it down with a warm beverage.

But what if you followed everything in the Hot Diet, except eliminating ice from drinks with your meals? Would that give you the weight loss you're seeking? Unfortunately, no, at least, it wouldn't in the long term.

In a 2004 study conducted by the Health and Social Care Information Centre in England, scientists followed a group of people who did everything right (meaning a balanced diet plus regular exercise), except (not knowing about the Hot Diet) they had ice with their drinks. They all gained weight. The results showed that obesity in that country had almost doubled in ten years, from 13.2 percent of the population in 1994 to 23.6 percent in 2004, despite the fact that the number of people exercising at least five times a week increased from 32 to 35 percent of men and 21 to 24 percent of women, and that the number of people eating at least five portions of fruit and vegetables each day actually increased. People were exercising more and eating a better diet, yet they still packed on the pounds.[6] It's not an isolated situation. Thousands of Americans who take care of themselves (according to commonly accepted standards) in terms of diet and exercise still struggle to achieve and maintain a healthy weight level. Even those people fortunate enough to have personal dietitians on their staff sometimes find it difficult to keep the weight off. Avoiding ice is the keystone. Without it, modest improvements in your diet and exercise programs just aren't enough to keep your weight within recommended ranges over the long run.

Remember, if you're consuming ice, you're crippling your metabolic efficiency. Ever so slowly, ice robs you of vital energy you need to keep moving and to build and maintain muscle mass. I can't repeat it often enough. *Ice is the poison that impedes even the best food, exercise, and lifestyle choices.* For long-term success, don't think you can shortchange the Hot Diet. Follow every element in it, especially the elimination of ice.

The Hot Diet, then, is actually very easy to follow:
1. Eat a balanced diet.
2. Eat in moderation, slowly and calmly.
3. Minimize stress in your life, especially at mealtimes.
4. Exercise.
5. Avoid ice.

One more thing: it may actually be safer to lose unwanted pounds slowly rather than faster. Try spreading your weight loss out over several months, never losing more than ten or twelve pounds in a single month.

So far I've told you everything about the Hot Diet except the specific foods it includes and how these help you lose weight. That will be covered in the next few chapters.

You can imagine how excited we were. This discovery had the potential to end mankind's diet problems forever. Millions of lives would be changed for the better. Countless hours of suffering from obesity-related diseases could be avoided completely. We were flying on top of the world.

Who would have guessed that just a few days later the Hot Diet would become the last thing on our minds as one of us suddenly looked into the face of death itself?

"You have to take care of this," the young doctor would say softly, "or two months from now, you may not be alive."

4: LIVING HOT

Fortunately for AJ and me, those haunting words of the young doctor were still somewhere off in the future, like a dark and distant storm barely visible over the horizon. Our days were being spent in growing excitement over sharing the Hot Diet with millions of people worldwide.

I was losing weight rapidly. I had gone through the full twenty-eight–day starter diet and now was on the maintenance diet. I was eating to complete satisfaction. Breakfast was now my largest meal of the day. Lighter lunches and even lighter dinners were causing me zero problems. I was never hungry.

No longer did I begin every meal with an ice-filled glass of soda. Instead, I was substituting hot tea, a drink I had not previously enjoyed. But it was now a vital part of every lunch and dinner, and I couldn't imagine how I had gotten along without it. The way it heated my insides felt warm and comforting. I had discovered that the Hot Diet was like no diet I had ever experienced before.

"*Diet* is a terrible word," AJ would say to me anytime I brought it up. "It conjures up images of fasting, deprivation, hunger, misery, and frustration."

The Hot Diet is none of those things. You won't be hungry, and you won't be miserable. It helps you make common sense decisions about the foods you eat. It also makes you conscious of the need for smaller (but more normal) portion sizes, the importance of regular exercise, and the benefits of reduced stress levels.

Before you begin any diet, of course, including this one, we strongly recommend that you consult with your physician for his or her approval before proceeding.

In this chapter, AJ goes in-depth to see exactly how you can start "living hot." Some of what he will discuss has been lightly touched on in previous chapters. It all bears repeating.

— **THE FIRST STEP IS TO ELIMINATE ICE FROM YOUR DIET. THIS** will not necessarily be easy, as the force of habit drives you to reach without thinking for that soda from the fridge and the ice from the freezer. That impulse will soon melt away, however, as you experience the advantages of warm fluids over cold.

Selecting foods on the Hot Diet is not so much a matter of which *individual* foods as it is which *combination* of foods. The Hot Diet does not recommend any one food over another. Instead, it emphasizes a good balance of the major food groups: meat, vegetables, fruits, and grains.

I studied whether certain foods might aid the body's metabolism better than others. Are there pro-metabolism "super foods" that actually improve the efficiency with which calories are converted into energy? The short answer is no. There are no magic foods that—just because you're eating them rather than an equally healthy alternative—let you eat your way to a lower weight. The body just does not work that way.

How many fad diets have fooled you with their far-out theories? "Magic" remedies have been tossed around in the form of herbal supplements, metabolism pills, cabbage diets, grapefruit diets, liquid diets, diet pills, herbal remedies, and in high protein/low carbohydrate, low protein/high carbohydrate food combination diets. All seriously miss the mark.

Your personal genetics, hormone levels, thyroid condition, diet history, lean body mass (muscle), amount of body fat, and even your ethnic background are the factors that determine your personal metabolic rate. The food you eat does not change that. One reason is that not everyone has the same metabolic rate—the speed at which your body burns calories. Some people have a very fast metabolic rate and tend to be quite slim. These people rarely become overweight. They're the people you love to hate at fancy parties or family reunions.

Others have a relatively slow metabolic rate and—without help—struggle with weight gain most of their lives.

How do you determine your own metabolic rate? The Basal Metabolic Rate (BMR) is a formula that calculates the number of calories your body requires while at rest to maintain normal bodily functions such as breathing, pumping your heart, maintaining your body temperature, and so forth. It indicates how fast your motor is running when you're in a reclined position or sleeping. Your metabolic rate can vary depending upon on your sex, how old you are, and how much muscle mass you have. Studies show that men have a 10 to 15 percent faster BMR than women because a larger percentage of their bodies is made of lean muscle tissues.[1] To calculate your personal BMR, use the following formula from the World Health Organization:[2]

WOMEN
65.5 + (4.35 x weight in pounds) + (11.7 x height in inches) −
(4.7 x age in years)
MEN
66 + (6.23 x weight in pounds) + (12.7 x height in inches) −
(6.8 x age in years)

Your BMI (Body Mass Index), on the other hand, is helpful not in defining whether you are or are not overweight, but whether you may *tend* to be overweight. If your BMI ranks in the overweight range, your amount of muscle mass will determine if you're considered overweight. Muscle weighs more than fat, therefore if you are muscular, you could have a high BMI but not necessarily be overweight according to this measurement. Another person with your BMI but far less muscle mass might be considered overweight.

You can measure BMI using the following formula:

$$\left(\frac{\text{Weight in pounds}}{\text{Height in Inches}^2} \right) \text{ X } 703$$

Here's the BMI table of values from the U.S. Department of

Health and Human Services, Center for Disease Control and Prevention:[3]

		CORRESPONDING WEIGHT IN POUNDS (APPROX.)	
Weight	BMI Values	Man 5'9"	Woman 5'4"
		(Avg. Height)	(Avg. Height)
Healthy Weight	18.5–24.9	121–163 lbs.	108–144 lbs.
Overweight	25.0–29.9	164–195 lbs.	145–173 lbs.
Obese	30+	196+ lbs.	174+ lbs.

A BMI greater than 25 may indicate that you are overweight. A BMI of 27.8 for men and 27.3 for women is the obesity cutoff point used by the National Health and Nutrition Examination Survey (NHANES II).[4] If your BMI is above those numbers, you're considered obese according to their standards. Once you determine your BMI and discover that it is too high, is there anything your food choices can do to help bring it down?

First, eliminate foods that provide poor fuel for your internal fire. Cut out sweets and candies that result in nothing but short bursts of energy—and long-term weight gain. Decide what you really want from life. Is it the momentary thrill of tasting something pleasant on your tongue—or is it a lifetime of health and energy? Look in the mirror, and if you can say you are 100 percent satisfied with the person looking back at you, at the way your clothes fit, at the energy you feel, then go right ahead and eat those foods you know you should avoid.

But if you prefer a trimmer version of your present self—a person with far more energy than you have today, a person less likely to suffer disease and disability in your future years—then start taking control today.

You can live fat, or you can live hot. It's your choice.

HOT DIET PRINCIPLE #1: EAT A BALANCED DIET

I studied everything the most respected nutritionists and health organizations in the world were saying about food and dieting. One that met my criteria for reliability and credibility is the Food Guide Pyramid, now called *MyPyramid*, from the U.S. Department of Agriculture. It is recommended by the American Dietetic Association, the U.S. Surgeon General, and the American Medical Association, among others.[5] Another good source of food recommendations is the Healthy Eating Pyramid created by nutrition experts at the Harvard School of Public Health. It bills itself as a refinement of the USDA Pyramid.[6] These are both excellent guidelines to a healthy diet. They include no fad foods, no excesses, and no surprises. They're a reminder that for countless centuries, man has been eating a naturally healthy diet and that it's time we returned to what history has proven to be successful.

In one sense, the foods on these pyramids are the nearly perfect Hot Diet foods. They all promote maximum efficiency in the digestive process.

WHOLE GRAIN FOODS

Grains are excellent sources of the carbohydrates needed for energy. They include whole wheat bread, brown rice, and oatmeal—all rich in energy-packed starches. One advantage of these grains is that the body cannot digest them as quickly as it does such highly processed carbohydrates as white flour. This tends to keep blood sugar and insulin levels at more moderate levels and reduces hunger pangs.

If your physician has determined that you have a poor tolerance for whole grain foods (containing wheat, barley, rye, or oats), you may want to drop this group from your diet and substitute gluten-free alternatives such as rice.

FRUITS AND VEGETABLES

These are some of nature's most beneficial foods, and the fact that they are so often ignored is an important indicator as to just how unhealthy our diets have become. Filled with critical vitamins and minerals, fruits and vegetables can be part of every meal or snack.

FISH, POULTRY, AND EGGS

This group provides the protein each of us needs. Fish, for example, is widely acclaimed for its ability to reduce the risk of heart disease. Poultry is a low-fat food that can be eaten alone or as part of countless other dishes. Eggs, once thought to contain high levels of cholesterol, are now considered to be key elements in a healthy diet—and a whole lot better with your morning breakfast than a doughnut or energy bar.

PLANT OILS

Harvard nutritionists found current evidence indicating that plant oils are good sources of healthy unsaturated fats. These fats improve cholesterol levels and protect the heart from potentially deadly rhythm problems. They include olive, canola, soy, corn, sunflower, peanut, and other vegetable oils as well as fatty fish such as salmon.

NUTS AND LEGUMES

Lace your diet with plenty of black beans, navy beans, garbanzos, and other dried beans, plus beneficial nuts such as almonds, walnuts, pecans, peanuts, hazelnuts, and pistachios. They are all very good sources of protein, fiber, vitamins, and minerals.

DAIRY PRODUCTS

Dairy products are excellent sources of calcium, which contribute to the formation of strong bones. Be careful, however, of the saturated fat in dairy products, not to mention the calories. Try no-fat or low-fat dairy products to keep the calories down. Better yet, take a daily calcium supplement. Forget the ice cream except on special occasions.

RED MEAT AND BUTTER

Americans eat too much red meat. In part, this may be due to fad diets of the past. Today we recognize that the amount of saturated fat in red meat makes it a food that should be eaten only occasionally. As an alternative, try fish or chicken to keep your cholesterol levels low. If you eat butter regularly, try going without—or switch to an alternate spread.

WHITE RICE, WHITE BREAD, POTATOES, PASTA, SWEETS

Eat these only sparingly. These foods can cause quick increases in blood sugar, resulting in weight gain, diabetes, heart disease, and worse. In fact, during your quick weight loss phase of the first several weeks or so, you may want to avoid these foods entirely. Potatoes, as suggested earlier, are an exception. Enjoy in moderation.

The reason I use the pyramid as part of the Hot Diet is that it promotes balanced consumption exceptionally well. If you make your food selection from the foods on this pyramid, you will satisfy the bulk of your nutritional needs. But remember, *moderation* is the key word in dieting. Eat none of these foods in excess.

After consulting with highly qualified nutritionists, I mapped out not only a recommended twenty-eight-day starting diet, but also a whole series of recipes using the foods of the pyramid as ingredients (see the chapters that follow).

The starting diet should contain no surprises for you. In addition to the USDA and the associations mentioned above, it follows the guidelines of the American Heart Association and even the American Cancer Association, both of which are strong advocates of a balanced diet. Remember, however, that balanced food selection is only part of the solution. Other elements may be just as important.

A diet in which food is not the most important factor? What kind of diet is this? It's the diet that no one else had come up with before. It has to be different. Nothing else has worked before.

Do you remember the five major principles of the Hot Diet?

1. Eat a balanced diet.
2. Eat in moderation, slowly and calmly.
3. Minimize stress in your life, especially at mealtimes.
4. Exercise.
5. Avoid ice.

We've just covered the first principle: Eat a balanced diet. But as we've discussed before, there's more to keeping your digestive fires burning efficiently than just monitoring the foods you eat.

BIG BREAKFAST, LIGHT LUNCH, LIGHTER DINNER

Perhaps you wonder if it makes any difference when we eat or how often. This is one of my most passionate areas of conviction.

We have already talked about the importance of starting your day with a healthy breakfast. But judging from the millions of people who ignore that advice, it bears repeating. Without food, you have no energy, especially in the morning when most of us haven't eaten for eight or ten hours or more. Yet there are people out there who will read this and think it doesn't apply to them. Why are they surprised when, either today or ten years from now, they look in a mirror and see an overweight person looking back? Breakfast is absolutely essential and not just a small breakfast either. Eat as if it's your main meal because that is what it should be.

By mid-morning, the average person is well into his daily activity. His body is craving energy, demanding it. So what do too many of us do? Very likely, we grab a donut or Danish for a quick energy rush. That's like throwing a thimble of gasoline on a fire. It flares up and in a few minutes is gone. No wonder you're extremely hungry at lunch or dinner.

If you make lunch your largest meal, you have only half a day to use up the calories you've consumed. It's even worse when you eat a large dinner. For most of us, the path from the dinner table to the couch is the only exercise we get once dinner is over.

This pattern has become commonplace only in the past forty years or so. Before that, breakfast was a main event, and few people skipped it. Lunch was called dinner, and dinner was called supper.

Parents back in the fifties and sixties would not have dreamed of skipping breakfast, and they certainly would not have allowed their children to do so. That changed during the "thin culture" of the seventies, eighties, and nineties. Along with breakfast bars and liquid meals came the concept that if you "saved calories" by missing breakfast, you were ahead in the weight game.

Nice try. But the body just doesn't work that way. Once the body realizes it isn't getting the food it needs, it tends to slip into a starvation mode. More calories are converted to fat—which is one way the body protects itself against anticipated lean times. The body says, "Hey, looks like we may be going into a period without food. Let's store up some fat to get us through the hard times."

When you do this day after day, is it any wonder you put on extra weight?

The Hot Diet, you will recall, stresses a nutritional start to the day. Don't cheat yourself by thinking you can get by with a hurried cup of coffee or an energy bar. Start your digestive fires burning with a healthy, well-balanced meal. Have a plate of sizzling hot bacon and eggs, for example, or maybe a slice of ham or sausage, a side of whole wheat toast, a glass of orange juice, and perhaps a cup of hot tea or cocoa.

Lunch should be your second heaviest meal of the day. Remember to avoid cold drinks. If you're eating fast food, take your time. Do not rush. Use your entire lunch hour (or however much time you're allotted) without rushing back to work. If you rush, you create unnecessary stress that actually impedes the digestive process. Eat slowly, and remember what your mother told you about chewing your food. I don't recall whether my mother said ten chews or twenty. But the idea of taking your time to let the digestive process begin in your mouth, not your stomach, was right on.

Dinner should be the lightest meal of the day. That's a complete reversal for many of us. The time from dinner to bedtime is relatively short, and usually a relatively inactive time, so we need fewer calories than we would at breakfast where the entire day stretches before us. Conventional wisdom says never eat anything after eight or nine o'clock in the evening. Hot Diet wisdom says never eat more than a fistful or so of food after six o'clock, including whatever you consume at dinner.

Should you become hungry in the evening or anytime during the day for that matter, eat a very light snack. Have hot tea (caffeine-free is best) to maximize your satisfaction with the snack.

You will eat less on this diet, yet you will find yourself having the most satisfying meal experiences of your life. When the world discovers the benefits of the Hot Diet's heavy breakfast, light lunch, and lighter dinner formula, huge changes can take place.

It's important that you keep your digestive fire going all day long, the way nature intended. Anthropologists tell us that our ancestors ate in small amounts as they grazed through the countryside. If they caught game, they cleaned it, cooked it, and ate it. If they came across fruit or vegetables growing in the wild, they didn't store them for later. They ate them on the spot. For countless generations, our digestive systems were accustomed to constant stimulation and gratification all day long.

But just as you would snuff out the fire at your campsite if you threw all the logs on too quickly, your digestive system also becomes less efficient when you feed it too much at one time. Let's take a closer look at Bill's experience as an example.

I have found AJ's advice to be right on target. Prior to the Hot Diet, my largest meal had always been dinner. After pushing back from the table, I more often than not ended up in front of the television, lacking the energy to do much more than occasionally raid the refrigerator. My snacks of choice were leftover desserts, usually accompanied by a cold soda.

Since the Hot Diet, however, dinner has become my lightest meal of the day. It typically consists of a cup or two of decaffeinated hot tea, a small portion of fish or meat about the size of a stacked deck of cards, some fruit, and a small amount of vegetables. Afterwards, I pour myself another cup of hot tea, and for another half hour or so, I enjoy the most wonderful feeling of contentment and satisfaction. Never am I hungry. Never do I feel the need for snacks a few hours after dinner. In fact, four or five nights a week I feel so energetic that I take a two- or three-mile walk.

HOT DIET PRINCIPLE #2: EAT IN MODERATION

— **EATING IN MODERATION IS ABSOLUTELY CRITICAL. M**ODERATION is key to keeping your body satisfied all day long. It keeps hunger pangs away and encourages you to remain faithful to your Hot Diet.

As stated previously, moderation is simply portion control.

My research showed that portion sizes have been growing steadily since the fifties and sixties, right along with waistlines. That's about the time that fast-food restaurants were becoming popular, taking huge bites out of the traditional customer base of sit-down restaurants.

Fast-food restaurants were quick to compete for market share, seeking to gain larger audience shares by offering larger and larger sandwiches and oversized servings of fries. Kids loved it, of course, and made fast-food restaurants their favorite places to eat. Few people paid any attention to the fact that Americans were stuffing themselves to death with enormous quantities of nutritionally suspect foods.

Sit-down restaurants were forced to compete for audiences they were losing to the fast-food giants. When a restaurant would have a grand opening to attract new patrons, it would offer larger and larger portion sizes. Steak houses built their reputations on the size of their meat servings. Salad bars became *All You Can Eat*. It was crazy, and it still goes on today.

From 1977 to 1998, the average soft drink grew in portion size from 13 fluid ounces/144 calories to nearly 20 fluid ounces/193 calories.[7] Cheeseburgers grew from 5.8 ounces/397 calories to 7.3 ounces/533 calories. Salty snacks that averaged 132 calories in 1977 were averaging 225 calories by 1998.[8]

If you're old enough, you may remember that three-inch bagels were standard twenty years ago. Today, they measure as many as six inches, with double the number of calories.

We're eating out more too. In 2005, Americans spent nine times more on eating out than they did thirty years earlier.[9] It was only during the past two decades that doggie bags became popular. Restaurants had reached the point that their portion sizes were larger than most people could comfortably finish in one sitting, so they had to take home the leftovers for their dogs.

If you take a doggie bag home, does your dog eat the leftovers—or do you?

Portions served at home are growing larger as well. The culture of *more is better* has found its way into the food packaging we bring home from the grocery store. Today, if we're not eating *man-size* portions—a nice way of saying *much larger portions*—some of us feel cheated. We fear that we are only setting ourselves up for hunger later if we don't stuff as much food into our stomachs as possible.

Not only that, but many of the larger portions we're eating are processed foods, not the healthier raw foods we used to eat. Processed foods rob our bodies of vital nutrients and vitamins. We're replacing quality with quantity, and that's just another of the many reasons our waistlines keep growing.

So how do you sever your addiction to larger portions?

Adding a warm beverage to your meal makes smaller servings much more satisfying than when you drink cold beverages. In fact, the warm beverage often makes it possible for you to be satisfied with portion sizes 50 percent smaller than you would otherwise consume.

As a guideline, I suggest limiting lunchtime and dinnertime serving sizes so that they never exceed the size of a man's folded fist—and that for the main entrée. Side dishes should be one-half to two-thirds of that. The entire meal should not leave you feeling like you overate. If it does, you probably did exactly that.

Remember that the stomach takes about twenty minutes to tell your brain that you've had enough. Don't keep eating until the hunger goes away. Eat moderately sized portions, and don't rely on your stomach to tell you when enough is enough.

Another good guideline: don't feel you have to finish everything on your plate. And don't force your children to finish everything on their plates. Every time you do, you're setting them up for adult obesity. A child who can't finish his plate is a child who has been served too much food. That makes you responsible, not your child.

All things in moderation, the saying goes. So it is with the Hot Diet.

HOT DIET PRINCIPLE # 3: MINIMIZE STRESS IN YOUR LIFE

One reason so many of us are overweight is that we run around helter-skelter in a near panic most of the time, meeting deadlines, moving kids from school to soccer and back, doing a thousand and one highly stressful activities. And then we come to the dinner table.

How can the digestive system work efficiently when stress levels are so high? It can't. Our stomach muscles cinch up from the stress. We eat too quickly. We pay little attention to our food or to food selection. We just want to get the meal over with and move on to the next train wreck. On top of that, we bring our troubles to the meal table with us. What is the single worst question you can ask at the dinner table?

Honey, how was your day?

That question is an invitation to chaos at your dinner table. For some reason, we all tend to talk about the worst things that happened to us during the day. As we fork in the potatoes and slosh down a beverage, we relive the horrible experience we had with the boss, with the idiot in shipping, with the client who never understands and always wants more for less.

The emotional side of eating is a frequently overlooked reason so many of us put on weight. In my thousands of observations of people eating in public venues, I noted a distinct relationship between those who were overweight or obese and those who were speaking in an obviously emotional, animated way.

Conversely, people who were trim or relatively trim often spoke calmly during their meals. They seemed to be enjoying their dining experience much more than others who used the occasion to let off steam. Minimizing stress when you eat is the spiritual side of dieting.

When you're feeling love, it has the added benefit of removing tension from the body. Food is more completely and efficiently processed when we are calm and loving. Stomach acids and enzymes are better able to complete their jobs. Ultimately, you get more from your food when you maintain a composed state of mind.

Play soft music in the background during a meal, rather than a blaring television. Silence is even better. A quiet, non-confrontational attitude between all participants in the meal is essential. I like to precede each meal with a short prayer or meditation, even if only for a moment or so. During that time, I thank the Creator who has blessed the earth with food, and all the people who helped bring it to my table.

Think of why we're here on the earth. As guests on this planet, we're here to live good and healthy lives. God never intended us to live in illness or pain because of problems with weight. That was a decision we each have made for ourselves.

We must recognize that we are not alone here. Our weight is sometimes a source of pain to others who worry about us or who are forced to help us because we cannot help ourselves. We have to make a positive decision to do something about it.

I often think about the role of food in my life as I meditate before a meal. I try to remember that it is a gift from God's bounty. I have a moral obligation to use it for my personal good and the good of everyone around me. If I have abused the food He gave me, I take personal responsibility for it, and I recognize that I cannot allow my weight problems to continue. God wants the best for me, and He will give me strength to achieve that, even if it means changing virtually everything about the way I live and the choices I make. God can do anything, and with His help, so can every one of us.

Be grateful for every meal, and wisely choose the food you

eat. Hippocrates, the father of medicine said, "Let food be your medicine and medicine be your food."[10]

HOT DIET PRINCIPLE #4: EXERCISE

Hot Principle Four is exercise. Learn to accept it: no successful diet ever worked for any length of time without a strong exercise component. As upright hominids, there's no way we can make our way safely through our journey on this planet without exercise. Consistent, vigorous exercise is an unavoidable part of developing and maintaining optimal body weight.

Go back to the example of the fire. What happens when you agitate a fire by stoking it? The flame grows brighter. Same thing when you exercise. Your digestive fire grows more efficient. You digest food more quickly and completely. Exercise assists in cleaning out your intestinal tract, prevents constipation, and helps you avoid many serious diseases attributed to inactivity.

Exercise is stoking your fire.

WALKING

Begin walking on the very first day of your Hot Diet. If you have not been in a walking regimen previous to starting this diet, begin by walking ten to fifteen minutes a day, five days a week (with your physician's permission, of course). Do this for two weeks, and then increase it to twenty minutes a day. Two weeks after that, increase it to thirty minutes. Keep increasing your walking minutes until you get up to at least forty-five minutes a day, four to five days a week.

Walk briskly. Do not stroll. Swing your arms as you walk

(that burns more calories), and maintain an upright body posture in which your chin is high and your back is straight. If exercise is the part of dieting you hate most, keep at it for at least four to six weeks, and it almost always becomes the part you like better than anything else.

Where can you walk? Almost anywhere. If the weather outside is bad, drive over to your local indoor shopping center and walk back and forth the entire length until your time is up.

Be like that guy I talked to in the Costco parking lot. Never drive when you can walk. Park plenty of distance from the door when you go shopping. Force yourself to take the long way. Avoid elevators and escalators you don't really need to take. Climb stairs. Join a walking club, or if there is not one near you, call up a couple of friends and start one.

FORMS OF EXERCISE

Other recommended forms of exercise include cycling, jazzercise, dancing, running, swimming, and more. Get involved with sports again. No matter what your age, you can find a sports activity that is ideal for giving you the exercise you need, and as an extra bonus, introduces you to new friends and enriches your life. Find something that gets you excited, and build it into your lifestyle.

Don't have time for walking or for playing a sport? Turn off the television. The average American spends hours in front of the television every day—and gets very little out of it. Back when there were only three channels, most of us got more exercise. But instead of blaming our obesity on the advent of multichannel cable, let's all just agree that we are still masters of our own TV remotes instead. Turn off your TV and live again!

Try getting up thirty minutes earlier. Buy a bicycle. Or if you absolutely must watch all that TV, do it while walking or running on a treadmill. The time is there; you just have to care enough to make room for it.

ANAEROBIC EXERCISE

Add some form of anaerobic exercise to your routine. The word *anaerobic* means *without air* and refers to the energy exchange that takes place in muscles during short high-intensity work-outs. Regain your youthful muscles.

Examples include weight lifting, sprinting, jumping—virtually any exercise that consists of short bursts of exertion (three minutes or so). The major benefit of anaerobic exercise is muscle building. Remember that muscles use calories all day long, so one of your primary goals on the Hot Diet should be to replace your current body fat with muscles like those you had in your twenties and thirties.

Start some type of anaerobic exercise immediately, going very slowly at first. Do fewer repetitions on lighter weights, increasing gradually as your body develops the muscles you're looking for. Work with your local health club personnel or hire a personal fitness counselor to guide you if you have not lifted weights before. Be careful, progress slowly, and you will soon see your arms beginning to take the kind of shape you've dreamed about. Your thighs will become trimmer and more compact, as will your entire body.

Soon you will no longer be embarrassed to show your arms

THE HOT DIET

and legs in public. Your waist will be trimmer. Your clothes will look better because they drape your body in a more complimentary way.

HOT DIET PRINCIPLE #5: AVOID ICE

The human body is amazing. There are more than twenty billion cells in our brain. Of these we use maybe one billion at the most. There are more than two hundred bones and almost seven hundred muscles. Sixty percent of the body is water, so it is very important to keep the temperature at an optimum level. It is vital to keep the digestive system warm and efficient.

Avoiding ice, as we have discussed throughout this book, can help you maintain maximum efficiency as you process food. Intellectually, this makes sense. Physically, it can make you thinner. Elimination of ice while eating is essential if you want to get off the dieting rollercoaster many Americans have been riding for as much as three decades. Your choices are simple: avoid ice and lose weight; consume ice and grow heavier.

The five principles of the Hot Diet can help you achieve your goals.

1. Use the best components—eat a healthy, well-balanced diet.
2. Preserve the fire—eat slowly and in moderation.
3. Keep pressure under control—minimize stress.
4. Stir the fire—exercise.
5. Optimize digestive temperatures—avoid ice.

When it comes down to it, the question is not whether you will have energy or not, but what are all the wonderful things you can do with this energy?

5: DETOUR

Who'd be calling me at seven in the morning?

I could hear the phone ringing as soon as I opened the door to my office. It was still early morning, a time when I like to get in before everyone else and answer waiting e-mails, check the news, or simply grab a moment of quiet before the rest of my office springs to life with activity.

The past couple of months had been busy. Not only was I losing weight on the Hot Diet, but AJ and I also had been making good progress toward putting it into book form. Our excitement was growing almost daily as we saw the enormous potential of the Hot Diet to solve weight problems. Best of all, my pants were fitting better. I was starting to lose the balloon-shaped figure that had been tailing me for a decade. I could look down at my sandals without seeing stomach before I saw toes.

I grabbed the phone from its cradle.

"Hello?"

It was AJ. There was a strange tone to his voice.

"Bill, I've got to talk to you. I haven't slept all night."

"What's the matter? What's going on?"

AJ reminded me of the physical he had scheduled for the previous afternoon.

"Well, they ran a whole battery of tests and . . ." he hesitated.

Suddenly I didn't like where this was going.

"I've got cancer, Bill."

You know that feeling when it seems as if a whole building is collapsing down around your shoulders? When you want to run somewhere and hide but can't because something is freezing you in place? AJ's words were sending cold shivers up and down my spine.

"Tell me what the doctors said, AJ. What kind of cancer? How bad?"

It was colon cancer, the same cancer that had killed my mother. My mind went back to a similar call I had received just a few years before. That's when I learned the tragic news about the woman who had raised, nurtured, and without reservation had loved my eight siblings and me. She was the matriarch of our family, the center of our activities—our cornerstone, our inspiration.

Diagnosed in February, she was gone by November.

Within a few minutes, AJ was in my office, and we were able

to talk face-to-face. I asked him to tell me all about it. He took a big breath and began to talk.

— IT SEEMS LIKE ONLY YESTERDAY THAT I WAS ON TOP OF THE world. My consulting trip to Japan had been a big success. Not only that, but in my quest to discover the answer to weight control, I was basking in the knowledge that I had finally solved the puzzle that had consumed me for the past five years.

But knowing it was time for my annual physical and because I had been having diarrhea since my return from Japan, I decided to set up an appointment with my primary physician. I figured the diarrhea was from eating too much sushi or from the stress of traveling, and a quick prescription would set me right again. Dr. Duda examined me thoroughly, commenting, "You're looking great for being fifty years old." For some reason, he suggested I visit Dr. Javaheri for a colonoscopy. "Always a good idea once you pass age fifty," Dr. Duda said.

Before I left, he took some blood samples, and a few days later, I was told the results were good. My diarrhea went away, and I continued my hectic traveling schedule. Following Dr. Duda's advice, I also made an appointment for the colonoscopy with Dr. Javaheri.

On the day of the procedure, I woke up early and took the dog for my usual five-mile walk on the trails close to our home. I love walking in nature. For me, it is always a rich experience of meditation, prayers, exercise, and the beauty of nature.

When I got to the hospital, I was directed to the left wing and two perky nurses greeted me: "Have you had a colonoscopy before?"

"No," I said nervously.

"Don't be nervous. Dr. Javaheri is very good and experienced. We have already done seven colonoscopies today. You'll be number eight."

"Wow, lucky me," I responded. "Isn't number eight lucky in Chinese?"

"I don't know," the redheaded nurse said. "I'm from Israel."

The doctor walked in.

"Go easy on me, doc," I said.

"You won't feel a thing."

I went into a nice sleep. An instant later it seemed, I was waking up to see tears in the eyes of both the doctor and his nurse. Something was wrong. The nice redheaded nurse touched my forehead as the doctor, taking a big breath, handed me the report.

"You definitely have cancer, AJ, and you must take care of it immediately. There is a polyp inside of you that has already grown thirteen centimeters, and it is invasive."

I said, "You've got to be kidding."

"No, AJ, this is very serious. I have already called an oncologist and a surgeon."

The kind nurse said, "Don't blame yourself. I will pray for you, but please take care of it immediately. We see a lot of men with colon cancer."

As I was being wheeled out of the hospital, I was in a daze of disbelief. Nevertheless, that night I went to my son's baseball game. Somewhere in the third inning, I leaned over to my wife and told her the news. I was trying desperately not to scare her, so I tried not to make a big deal out of it. I didn't fool her for a second.

The next day, I visited an oncologist. Dr. Wagner ordered more tests to see what stage my cancer was in. He told me the colonoscopy was accurate and that I definitely had colorectal cancer.

How could this have happened to me? There had been almost no signs. Why, I had been at the peak of fitness, walking more than four miles several times a week if not daily. I left younger men huffing and puffing behind me when we walked together.

Shortly after the colonoscopy, I showed the report to Dr. Joe Ruggio, a neighbor who is a prominent heart surgeon. He told me what I'd been hearing over and over: that my case didn't look good and that I should take care of it immediately. He made an appointment for me with Dr. Rod, a colorectal surgeon.

"He's one of the best," Dr. Ruggio said. "It's hard to get an appointment with him, but because he's a friend and because of the urgency, he's agreed to see you tomorrow morning. Don't put this off, AJ. It's very serious."

Like the others, Dr. Rod read the report and examined me. "AJ, everything your other doctors have been telling you is true. You need to drop everything and take care of this right now. Otherwise, in two months you may not be here. Go and get a CAT scan immediately. Let's hope the cancer hasn't spread to the other parts of your body, especially the liver."

I learned later that a CAT scan is a process in which a computer takes data from multiple X-ray images and turns them into pictures on a screen. CAT, which stands for Computerized Axial Tomography, reveals soft tissue structures that are invisible in conventional X-rays. Using about the same dosage of radiation as an ordinary X-ray machine, the CAT scan shows individual slices of the body with extreme clarity.

I went in for the CAT scan, and by the time I finished, it was 3:00 p.m. and a beautiful day outside. I was hoping for the best but knew somehow that the CAT scan would only confirm what all these experts had been telling me. Looking up at the soft white clouds and blue sky overhead, I whispered a silent prayer to God to protect me, so small and vulnerable in His vast universe.

The next day I got another opinion. That doctor, too, looked at the CAT scan report and, like the others, began to shake his head.

"Your case is very advanced," the doctor said. "The polyp is around ten years old and has been cancerous for possibly four years. The CAT scan also shows some spots on your liver. The tumor has grown and has gone through the intestine, and because it is located very low and deep, very few doctors can operate on it."

My chances, he was saying, were slim or none. It was a stage four cancer, the most advanced kind. He gave me anywhere from two months to two years to live. Looking over at my wife, who had accompanied me, the doctor said, "You may want to spare him from the pain of surgery."

It was more than I could stand. The anger was welling up inside me and began to spill out: "Lance Armstrong was stage four, and he is cancer free! By God's will, I will beat it too!"

Gently, the doctor laid his hand on my arm. "That's wishful thinking, I'm afraid. Besides, Armstrong had testicular cancer. There are 102 known cancers. Colon cancer, when as far along as yours, is usually fatal, AJ."

I don't remember much about the trip home. But I do know it was a terrible evening at our house. When the kids heard the news, they began to cry softly. Slowly the realization was taking hold, and the questions were pouring out. Are we going to keep our home? Would we have to move to an apartment or a town-house? What would happen to us, to them? Is Dad going to die?

I could feel the cold tentacles of fear inching their way up my spine and weaving themselves in and about my innermost organs, down where my spirit lives. Was that fear I was feeling? Or just weakness? I was conscious of a growing pain in my stomach. Somewhere deep inside me, a small voice warned that if I surrendered, if I let the fear take over, the disease would grow faster.

I hesitated to tell people outside of my immediate family. I had to be sure first. Facing death was new to me. You never know how you'll respond until it happens to you. That night in bed, I watched my entire life parade in front of me. I thanked God for the good things with which He had blessed my family and me. "Thank you for the gift of life You have given me. I am grateful, and if You want to take me, I'm ready. But I know this is a test, and You want me to overcome it, so I can be stronger in serving you."

A short while later something out of the ordinary hap-pened. I may have been sleeping, or I may have been awake; I don't know. I do know I felt someone—was it an angel, a spirit?—touching my stomach at the site of my deepest pain, saying, "You will be okay."

I awoke with a strength that I had never felt before, a determination that seemed to fill every pore in my body. I started calling my family and friends, urging them to get a colonoscopy, saying it may be too late for me, but it could save your lives. That was the best thing I did because in return I got great advice from some, along with many kind words of support.

So how would I handle this incredible disaster that had come into my life? Suddenly, as had happened back when I decided to begin my study of the causes of obesity, I remembered the words of Abraham Lincoln: "The best way to destroy your enemy is to make him your friend."[1]

Cancer is a terrible enemy. Like a terrorist, it was terrorizing my family and me. I learned that, according to the American Cancer Society, more than 106,000 people get colon cancer every year, and nearly 42,000 are diagnosed with rectal cancer. Colorectal cancer was estimated to account for more than 55,000 deaths in 2006.[2]

Approximately half of the colorectal patients survive their disease.[3] So then and there I made the determination to be a survivor. I figured if I received the best treatment, the statistics would be in my favor. I was not going to surrender to fear. I felt comforted knowing that God gives us strength we don't even know we have. He has a plan for each of us.

So I switched into an action mode. I learned that the University of Southern California (USC) has one of the most respected cancer centers in the U.S. My contacts told me that if I could just get an appointment with USC's Dr. Robert Beart, I might have a better chance of surviving this cancer. With the help of friends and family, I was able to get an appointment quickly. Dr. Beart examined me and immediately ordered a PET scan, which showed that the liver and the other organs were clear, but the lymph was questionable.

AJ's illness changed everything. The pages that I had been knocking out so quickly soon slowed to a snail's pace as his attention turned to his treatment. He traveled to Los Angeles every day as the chemotherapy portion of his treatment began. The doctors put him on chemo for eight weeks and combined chemo and radiation treatment for six weeks following that. Early on in the treatments, he looked amazingly healthy and robust. A stranger would not have known he was suffering a life-threatening disease. His spirits were invariably high as he called me almost daily.

"Bill, how goes the book?" he'd ask. "I'll fight the cancer; you write that book!"

I'd sit down at the computer to write but found it difficult to make headway. The thought of what AJ and his family were enduring took a toll on the great excitement I had had for the project. Like AJ, I also turned to prayer. I called on a good friend, an internationally known Catholic mystic, to keep AJ in her prayers. She in turn contacted others to pray for him. Many others, Christian and non-Christian alike, also remembered AJ in their prayers.

What we did not see, of course, was the pain and turmoil that AJ's family endured. Anyone who has had cancer knows that the hardest path is often the one traveled by the patient's family. AJ's wife and children, relatives, and friends were all drawn together as they found their loved one apparently on the brink of eternity.

The only way I could help AJ was to keep writing. Slowly, as his treatment continued, the chapters of the Hot Diet book were coming together. As AJ was always reminding me, weight problems around the world would not go away just because he had cancer.

"Just write," he would plead with me over the phone. In the background I could hear the mechanical beeps and clicks of medical equipment hooked up to his body to monitor his condition. Every now and then, he had to pause a moment to catch his breath or to wait for the pain to go away.

He never lost hope.

"Bill, I am determined not to lose my hair!" AJ kept saying. In the cancer center, he had witnessed other patients losing their hair. Some were devastated by it. Others made the best of it and wore brightly colored scarves and hats. AJ soon became known as the patient with the never-fading smile—nurses teased him about it—and he kept all of his hair.

Toward the end of the first eight weeks of chemotherapy, it was evident that he was being physically drained. The harsh chemicals were having their effect. His smile gradually became weaker, and he no longer had that energetic bounce in his step. The disease was pushing him to his limits.

After the chemotherapy and the subsequent six weeks of radiation, the doctors informed him that the polyp had finally begun to shrink. Four months after the initial diagnosis, surgeons removed the polyp and took a closer look at his internal organs. They discovered what the films could not show: the lymph was indeed infected, and it, too, was removed. The biopsy indicated the presence of some live cancer cells, so AJ was put on four more months of chemo-therapy.

This was the hardest part of his journey. The recovery turned out to be slower and more painful than he had antici-pated—the surgeons had to go deep inside his body to make the proper excisions, they said. So as he began that second round of chemo, he found himself suffering from the deep pains of the surgery as well.

Six months later, AJ underwent surgery again, this time to put his colon back together. And then one day, it was all over. No more chemo or radiation. No more surgery. The cancer appeared to be gone. AJ had joined the fifty-three thousand survivors who beat colon cancer every year.

"You can't say I'm cured yet," he told me. "Doctors don't claim a cure for at least five or ten years after the treatment is over. Every day I get up and thank God for giving me the day, I offer Him my suffering and ask Him to be with me. I get great pleasure spending every day with God."

THE HOT DIET AND CANCER

— COULD THE HOT DIET HAVE BEEN IN ANY WAY RESPONSIBLE for my cancer? I had been on the Hot Diet for almost six months before my cancer was discovered. Was there something terribly wrong with the Hot Diet, something we had never considered? I asked my doctor if the Hot Diet could be a fac-tor, and he assured me that because my polyps were almost ten years old and had been actively cancerous for perhaps four years, the Hot Diet had nothing to do with it.

In fact, when the doctors gave me a sheet of diet tips—the same sheet they give every patient—I immediately scanned the list of recommended foods and lifestyle suggestions (regular exercise, avoidance of stress, etc.) that the American Cancer Society recommended for cancer patients.

Number seven on the list was "Avoid ice water."

It blew me away. Had the American Cancer Society known the secret of the Hot Diet? Did they understand how ice water negatively affected the digestive process? Was there some kind of cover-up going on?

Such was not the case, I soon discovered. My doctor said that ice and ice water sometimes aggravate certain side effects of chemotherapy, so they simply recommend that patients avoid it. In fact, for other side effects such as dry mouth, patients are commonly urged to suck ice chips to relieve the dryness.

Today, I have returned to full health. Why did God choose to throw me this curve?

At one time, I wondered if the cancer episode was the price I had to pay for discovering the Hot Diet breakthrough. I mean, I had received something of enormous value from the universal treasury of wisdom as it were, something that could save thousands of lives around the world. Was there a price to be paid?

I knew, of course, that God doesn't work that way. Rewards in life, like obstacles, are just that and nothing more. Enjoy them when you receive them. I also learned that the true value of an obstacle such as cancer is the courage and strength we are forced to find within ourselves as we struggle to overcome it. The realization that life's hardships help us grow into stronger persons is reward in and of itself.

I soon realized that my personal experiences might be of use to other cancer patients. Research shows that cancer is preventable in many cases if only people would pay closer attention to their diets. We cannot allow ourselves to continue to abuse our bodies with too much of the wrong kind of food. We cannot lead sedentary lives. I had been focusing purely on obesity and the problems it causes, but God has reminded me in a very clear way that we have many more reasons to watch our diets.

Cancer is a great plague inflicting immense suffering and death on mankind, and it remains largely unconquered. It seems like only yesterday that President Nixon declared war on cancer. That was more than thirty years ago. Today, cancer is still one of the top three killers of Americans, along with heart and circulatory diseases. Virtually every family in the country is affected by cancer in one way or another. Tragically, many of these deaths are preventable through proper diet, exercise, and regular physical examinations. It is important to look for the seven danger signals of cancer. Consult your physician immediately if you have any of the following:[4]

- Any sore that does not heal
- A lump or thickening in the breast or elsewhere
- Unusual bleeding or discharge
- Any change in a wart or mole
- Persistent indigestion or difficulty in swallowing
- Persistent hoarseness or cough
- Any change in normal bowel habits

In 2005, more than 7.6 million people died of cancer world-wide. Colon cancer alone resulted in 665-thousand deaths annually.[5]

Among the many medical professionals at the USC Department of Colorectal Surgery who worked with me was a particularly engaging and proficient nurse named Yolee Casagrande. During the course of my treatment, Yolee helped answer my many questions. She explained how polyps in the colon are abnormal growths much like moles on the skin. Almost one in three persons has such colorectal polyps at age fifty, she told me, and at age eighty almost 55 percent of us have them. Polyps can grow over a long period of time—approximately ten years—before some of them turn cancerous.[6]

That's why physicians often recommend polyp screening every ten years beginning at age fifty (age forty-five for African American patients), and sometimes even more frequently if your family history dictates it. Your physician may also recommend flexible sigmoidoscopy tests every five years and fecal occult blood tests (FOBT) every year.[7] If you have any questions about polyp screening, be sure to consult your personal physician.

Today, months after my early morning phone call to give Bill the bad news, we have a new appreciation of the importance diet plays in our lives. What was it about my diet ten years ago that may have led to the formation of that first tiny polyp in my colon? Were there other causes or circumstances leading to the cancer? Hereditary causes? Environmental? Pure chance?

We had learned that eternity is never more than a heartbeat away. Today could be the last day of life for any one of us, but we definitely do impact the direction our lives take. The foods we eat, the activities we partake in, and the lifestyles we lead all determine our futures upon this planet. The cancer opened my eyes to what is important in life. This is not the book that we had spent so much time planning. When man plans, God smiles.

6: BEYOND FOOD

In the weeks and months following AJ's recovery from cancer, he found his research into the causes of obesity was gradually leading him into areas he had not considered before. His brush with death seemed to have lifted a veil from his eyes, and he began to consider the following new, previously unexplored aspects of weight control.

THREE COMPONENTS TO WEIGHT GAIN AND FAILED DIETS

— I THOUGHT THAT WE HAD NAILED IT BACK BEFORE MY ILL-ness. The five Hot Diet principles cover every aspect of the chemical process of digestion, everything from balancing food selection and portion control to regular exercise and avoiding ice. But then, in the middle of the emotion and trauma over my bout with cancer, I suddenly realized that weight gain and failed diets had more than a biochemical component. I discovered that there are actually three components in all: (1) biochemical, (2) emotional, and (3) spiritual.

THE BIOCHEMICAL COMPONENT

The biochemical component is implemented through the five principles of the Hot Diet as laid out in Chapter Three. Other diets may have one or more of these principles, but only the Hot Diet includes the critical avoidance of ice.

The Hot Diet is the first diet to treat the body as a machine. Applying mechanical chemistry to biochemistry as it relates to the digestive process works very well. But the body is much more than a machine.

THE EMOTIONAL COMPONENT

If we want our bodies to serve us efficiently, we have to look at everything that affects weight gain. There is another critical component of dieting—over and above the mechanical or biochemical—that contributes to successful dieting.

That component is emotion.

Consider the role emotion plays. It's almost impossible to lose weight when you're drowning in negative emotions. Millions of people have tried diet after diet without success because they fail to recognize how emotions affect their willingness to eat healthy foods, to control serving portions, or to exercise. I believe we have to consider three groups of emotions:

1. Love, compassion, understanding
2. Fear, anxiety, worry
3. Anger, hatred, rage

Positive emotions—love, compassion, understanding—tend to bring order to your eating habits. You eat more slowly; you don't gorge yourself. But when you're feeling a negative emotion—fear, anxiety, worry, anger, hatred, rage, and so forth—it's more comforting to stuff yourself with boxes of potato chips, candy, or sugar than it is to eat sensible portions of properly balanced meals or to take a brisk thirty-minute walk around the neighborhood.

Negative emotions can actually affect your waistline as much as they affect your attitude. Think about how often you've experienced this. You felt depressed, so you raided the fridge for a piece of cake. You felt sad, so you reached for a box of junk food. You felt stress, so food was your stress reliever. The mind/body connection is not just a theory—it is a reality.

An estimated 30 percent of all people who seek treatment for serious weight problems have tendencies toward binge eating. Studies have shown that emotions such as anger, anxiety, discontent, boredom, and sadness can lead people to find comfort in food.[1] Major events such as losing a job, a pet, or even an argument with a spouse lead many people to seek release in the food pantry or refrigerator. Eating becomes an obsession, an escape, and slowly the results show up as increased weight. That only adds to their other problems, so they enter a vicious whirlwind from which there is no exit. More food leads to more weight. More weight leads to more food.

When our emotions turn negative, dieting becomes incredibly more difficult. After you've started a new diet, how many times have negative emotions turned you back to comfort food? Were you feeling deprived because of the food you were giving up—and more than a little bit sorry for yourself? Were you comforting yourself after an argument, a rejection by a loved one, or a sudden drop in self-esteem? If you are not at peace within yourself, you cannot live in the atmosphere of calm, peace, and joy that the body needs to operate efficiently.

When stressed from a hard day of raising kids or troubles at work, how many times have you grabbed a soda or some other beverage out of the fridge and poured it into an ice-filled glass, seeking to soothe the churning turmoil inside your stomach? In its earliest uses, ice often served as an anesthetic. People found that rubbing it over aching bones and joints numbed the body's sensitivity to pain. So it's not surprising that for some people, icy beverages seem to numb their painfully knotted-up stomachs. The truth is, ice numbs vital chemical-producing cells along the lining of the stomach. The extreme cold shuts them down and slows their release of digestive fluids even if only for a short time until the body temperature can again rise to normal levels. Negative emotions actually change the efficiency of the digestive process, making weight problems harder to overcome when compared to people who have their emotions under control, who don't let things such as stress and anger gain the upper hand.

Uncontrolled negative emotions manifest themselves in ugly pounds that attach themselves to our stomachs, thighs, hips, and buttocks. Gaining control of our emotions, therefore, is an important part of losing weight.

THE SPIRITUAL COMPONENT

The spiritual dimension of our lives is a third necessary component of a good diet program. The respect we have for our bodies—because they were given to us by the Creator—can actually prompt us to stop the damage done by irresponsible eating and drive us to take charge of our personal health needs.

We are all temporary guests upon this earth, graced by God with a temporal body that is ours to use during our stay here. Clearly it is up to us as guests to ensure that our bodies remain healthy.

Excessive eating may actually violate our God-given responsibility to care for our bodies. Obesity, where controllable (meaning it is not caused by some other physical condition), could be looked at as a sign that we are not treating our bodies with the respect that God intended. Again, I'm talking about situations where a person can control his weight, not a situation where uncontrollable illnesses or circumstances are causing the weight gain.

As noted previously, obesity leads to many different types of illnesses, consumes many financial and natural resources, and extracts a heavy toll on our loved ones. Isn't there some sort of debt piled up when we wreak such havoc upon our fellow visitors and upon the environment?

Are we not answerable to God when, through thoughtless or deliberate overeating, we damage the vessels in which He placed our souls? Don't we have a responsibility for polluting the earth with garbage dumps full of processed food boxes, soda cans, and much more, including all those worn-out refrigerators oozing with dangerous ozone-damaging Freon?

Of course we do. But how many of us, sitting there in our soft chairs, slowly eating ourselves to death on calorie-rich snacks washed down with iced sodas, ever think about it? We have a duty to be good guests on this earth, remembering at the same time that we share the earth with other creatures of God. Ultimately we must all answer to God for the way we do or do not respect our bodies and the planet.

If you don't think excessive eating habits are endangering this planet, just look at all the waste dumps filled with discarded food wrappers that will still be there fifty years from now. Better yet, look at all the homes with a second refrigerator or freezer. That's where we keep all the frozen foods we've become addicted to. It's estimated that thirty-two million homes have a second fridge or freezer. What is the reason for that? If we were eating in moderation and treating our bodies with respect, would we need extra refrigerators? Would we need all that Freon that will inevitably find its way to our garbage dumps? Of course not. Get rid of excessive, energy-wasting refrigerators and freezers.

Refrigerators built before 1994 are a special concern because they contain levels of chlorofluorocarbons (CFCs) that can potentially damage the ozone layers. Two different types of CFCs are used in the manufacture of refrigerators. The first is CFC-11, used as a blowing agent in producing polyurethane insulating foam in the refrigerator. The other is CFC-12, used as a refrigerant in cooling circuits. Since 2003, all new refrigerators and freezers have been manufactured without ozone-depleting substances. The problem lies with the older, more dangerous refrigerators and freezers still running in many home basements and garages.

How many barrels of oil are consumed every day just to keep those old refrigerators operating? The real energy crisis may be in our basements and garages.

OTHER COSTS

There are countless other costs to overeating: Hospitals spending billions of dollars a year treating diabetes, heart ailments, and cancer—common results of overeating and obesity. The time invested by family and friends who change their lives to care for us. Bigger grocery bills. Higher clothing costs (multiple wardrobes to handle our changing sizes). Lost relationships as spouses lose attraction to their mates. Social ridicule as people snicker at our bulging bellies, ponderous thighs, and swaying cabooses.

Worst of all is the cost to ourselves as we struggle with sagging self-esteem and depression. We have a moral obligation to take responsibility for our bodies and for our health.

INCORPORATING THE EMOTIONAL AND SPIRITUAL COMPONENTS

So how do we incorporate the emotional and spiritual into the Hot Diet? Of the two, the emotional component may be the more challenging. That's because it is the more complex. The renowned psychoanalyst Sigmund Freud used to say there are three strong emotions: love, fear, and anger. My theory is that when it comes to our weight problems, it is not just emotions that count but the conflict between them.

- Love , compassion, understanding versus

- Fear, anxiety, worry versus

- Anger, hatred, rage

Various emotions create chemical changes in the body. For example, when we feel anger or hatred, our pulse rates speed up. Our faces become red and our blood pressure spikes up. The adrenal gland pours extra adrenaline into the blood stream, preparing the body in case a fight occurs. These are body mechanisms learned after millennia of human development—from the time when man hunted large beasts near his cave to the present time when we encounter the beast in people all around us. Our bodies have learned that hatred and anger are followed by certain events, and they have learned to adjust their internal mechanisms to survive.

Fear and anxiety evidence similar changes in the body. We may start shaking and trembling. We may feel dizzy or appear pale. Somehow we're weaker, more vulnerable. Out of self-preservation, we sometimes feel the need for flight.

Under either of these two conditions, fight or flight, avoid eating if at all possible—not that it would even occur to you. That's because when the body feels stress, it begins to release cortisol, a hormone secreted by the adrenal glands that, when released into the bloodstream, does any number of things. Before we get to the "bad" things, here are the "good" effects of cortisol:

- Regulation of glucose metabolism

- Regulation of blood pressure

- Regulation of insulin for blood sugar maintenance
- Regulation of the immune function
- Regulation of the inflammatory response

Some people call cortisol the *stress hormone* because of its powerful role during the body's fight-or-flight response to stress. From the above list, you can easily see the positive effects of cortisol. It generates a quick burst of energy that can be absolutely critical when a saber-toothed tiger is nipping at your heels—or when a mugger is bearing down on you in a dark stairway. It can sharpen memory functions, temporarily boost immunity, reduce sensitivity to pain, and help maintain homeostasis in the body. That's all good.

Unfortunately, cortisol also generates potentially negative responses. Foremost among them is that in stress conditions cortisol can instruct the body to store belly fat. This may be a throwback to prehistoric days when stress went hand-in-hand with scarce game in the forests or a paltry harvest in the fields. The body learned that the more belly fat you had, the better your chances of living through the winter. Today, however, most health experts recognize that excess belly fat is more dangerous to health than fat stored in other parts of the body. Some of the problems associated with belly fat are strokes, heart conditions, higher levels of LDL cholesterol (that's the bad kind), and lower levels of HDL cholesterol (the good kind).[2]

Cortisol also causes nasty conditions such as suppressed thyroid function, blood sugar imbalance, cognitive impairment, higher blood pressure, decrease in muscle tissue and bone density, and more. Not all of us, fortunately, experience the same results from cortisol secretion. Some of us react to stress differently than others. In the exact same stress situations, one person may secrete higher levels of cortisol than someone else. People who secrete these higher levels often eat more food, especially food higher in carbohydrates. If you're among those who are sensitive to stress and if you believe that stress may be one of the causes of your weight gain, it's critical that you learn stress management techniques and adjust your lifestyle to eliminate unnecessary stress.

My advice is simple: *at all times, practice love and understanding.* Love and understanding are critical not only in order to live a happy, stress-free life but also to achieve long-lasting dieting success that endures a lifetime.

But how do you eliminate the stress you may be bringing to the dinner table? How do you banish negative emotions such as hatred and anger or fear and anxiety just as you're about to sit down to a meal?

I observed so many people in my research who had obviously brought negative emotions to the table with them. Some were angry, some were upset. None of them were enjoying their meal, and probably none had any idea how their emotions were stimulating harmful cortisol production within their bodies.

It is much better to approach every meal with great calm and peacefulness. Recognize that meals should be times of love and understanding. Spend a few quiet moments before you begin to either prepare the food or to eat. Think about the gift that God has given you through this food. Be grateful to the farmer who planted and harvested the wheat seeds. Thank God for the rain He sent to soak the fields. Send warm thoughts of gratitude to the baker who mixed the batter and baked the loaves. Think kindly about the truck driver who moved the grain from farm to factory and store. Bless the stock persons and clerks who made your visit to the store convenient and pleasant. Bless the cook.

If you are eating with others, link hands with them as you thank God for the food He has given your family. The earth produces so much bounty, yet some unfortunates do not enjoy the bounty that you do. Pray for them too.

Be thankful for all who have touched the food before you, for all who had a hand in its placement before you. Food is a gift, and it is right that we express gratitude to those who have given it to us. Be thankful for the great variety and bounty of the earth itself.

You say you've always been grateful for such things? Good— then you will have no problem with the Hot Diet suggestion that before eating, you take a moment or two and shift into a reflective mode, to calm your body and collect your thoughts.

In the process, you will find that your stress is melting away. Your biochemistry is changing from fear and anxiety or anger and hatred to love and compassion. Your body no longer senses the survival crisis brought on by stress. It feels no need to produce cortisol, so more of your food goes to energy and less to stored fat.

Before you begin your meal, make sure you turn off the television and the stereo. Turn off your cell phone too. These are distractions that can add unnecessary tension to your meal, so eliminate them. Soft, gentle music playing in the background can add immensely to the experience.

Imagine that your dinner companion is a very important person. What would you say to that person? How would you behave? What would be your manner? Courteous? Respectful? Placid? That should be your demeanor no matter who joins you at the table, but especially if it is your family.

Many people have told me they'd like to have dinner with Jesus. Actually, we do that every day, don't we, whether we see Him or not? We are guests of the Creator because He provided food no matter how we acquired it. Decide today to eat slowly and respectfully at all meals, even the smallest ones. If you follow this practice, I can almost guarantee that you will discover a mealtime pleasure and contentment you have not experienced in years.

Begin your meal with a warm beverage or warm soup.

Again, eat slowly, constantly reminding yourself how special this meal is. Chew your food well. Give the digestive process time to begin in your mouth, as nature intended, not in your stomach. If others are at the table with you, remind yourself how fortunate you are to have their company. One day they may not be available to you, and you will regret not enjoying them while you could.

Keep all conversations calm, peaceful, and joyful. Allow no arguments, disagreements, or negative comments. Say nothing that will lead the conversation into a negative direction.

Your food, of course, should be that already recommended for the Hot Diet. Eat plenty of vegetables and raw fruits. There are no forbidden foods on the Hot Diet. Avoid ice and very cold dishes, being content in the knowledge that they are the poisons that caused your weight gain and that you can live perfectly well without them. If you absolutely must have a cold salad (great for adding fiber and roughage to your diet), eat it last.

Calories, by the way, *do* count. When you consume more calories than your body needs for energy, you will inevitably gain weight. Be in control of portion sizes. Many people on the Hot Diet report that they are able to cut their calorie intake significantly below what they used to consume just by having a warm beverage with each meal. The warm beverage allows them to be satisfied with much smaller portions. Remember that food is fuel for your body and that your body is a sophisticated mechanism. It will tell you when it has had enough fuel for the day. When it does, stop eating.

Make the warm beverage with every meal your visible commitment to living a thinner, more natural life. Many Hot Dieters report that after completing dinner, they like to take a warm cup of tea into their living room or TV room and leisurely sip the beverage as they relax and the meal is being digested. This greatly extends the pleasure of the meal, especially if it was one of minimal portion sizes as recommended by the Hot Diet's dinner suggestions.

Rarely are Hot Dieters hungry later in the evening. You will find that drinking a warm beverage during and after the meal is highly instrumental in helping you to avoid significant weight gain during the next few months and in keeping it off for the rest of your life. If you habitually skip the warm beverage, your chances of success may be diminished.

As I was planning this book, I argued with myself as to whether a chapter on the emotional and spiritual aspects of dieting really belonged. What if someone did not share my belief in God? But I had become convinced that what drives a person to gain weight is not just hunger. In fact, it is often something entirely different, something emotional in nature. I also realized that a truly successful, permanent solution had to be anchored in a higher purpose, such as the conviction that there are moral reasons to care for the bodies that God has given us.

My close experience with death made me realize how important it is to be grateful not only for life but also for an awareness of God as Creator. Each of us has been made unique. We have a duty to take care of these unique machines we live in, our bodies, and to help others realize how much work God has put into creating our individuality. We need to recognize our potentially positive impact upon our fellow travelers on this planet, including ways we can make their journeys more pleasant. We need to share the love God has put in each of us and not let that love turn to fear, hatred, or other negative emotions and feelings, all of which have a negative impact on our bodies.

The flame of the Hot Diet burns best when it burns pure, so we need to recognize our responsibility to achieve balance and simplicity—not only in our eating habits but also in our emotions, our spiritual convictions, and our treatment of others.

Balance keeps the universe in harmony. Without balance, our individual existences slowly go awry. We lose control. We injure ourselves and others. We disrupt the calm necessary for order in our lives. And with a certainty that is astonishing, we gain weight.

With the addition of emotional and spiritual balance, the Hot Diet is now complete.

7: AMERICA'S OVERWEIGHT CHILDREN

As AJ and I discussed overweight children, I shared a story from my grade-school experience. There was just one obese child in my small class of twenty-five or so students. We'll call her Mary (not her real name), and to my classmates, she was the butt of all the jokes. Mary was constantly referred to as *Fatso* or *Whale Butt* or equally hurtful names. When teams were picked, she was the last chosen. When the fifth grade recess mob rampaged throughout the schoolyard looking for a victim, she was the first they cornered. No one wanted to sit next to her in the classroom or auditorium.

Only as an adult did I wonder what our thoughtless,

adolescent behavior must have done to poor Mary. How many tears had we caused?

Mary's mom had a weight problem, too, as did her two sisters. Had we given it any real thought, I suspect we would have realized Mary's obesity could have come from any number of causes, including everything from medical conditions to family environment or lack of self-esteem.

Unfortunately for Mary, our childhood was a time when obesity was rare. Mary's weight made her stand out like a plump thumb. Today, however, she would have fit right in. Childhood obesity has become a national epidemic in America. In classrooms across the nation, there are many Marys. The number of overweight children aged six to nineteen almost tripled between 1976 and 2004.[1]

AJ's research into obesity started with the realization that his son was adding pounds over and above the norm for other children his age. What AJ learned about childhood obesity alarmed him.

AJ'S WAKE-UP CALL

— I HAD NO IDEA THINGS WERE GETTING SO CRITICAL UNTIL ONE day, shortly after noticing that my son John was packing on the pounds, I was relaxing on the patio, thinking about the neighborhood where I grew up. I remembered the sounds of kids playing, kicking the ball around, chasing each other in one kind of game or another, the noise of their games floating over the fences and throughout the neighborhood. But where were those noises today? The weather was perfect, school was out, but all I heard were birds. What had happened to the sounds of kids playing?

Searching for my son, I found him slouched in a chair in his room, deeply absorbed in some kind of computer game. "Why aren't you outside playing?" I asked.

"Because that's not as much fun as this game," John responded. "I just don't feel like running around today."

I knew I had a problem on my hands.

According to a 1999–2000 survey conducted by the National Health and Nutrition Examination Survey (NHANES), an estimated 16 percent of children and adolescents ages six to nineteen years are overweight.[2] Compare all NHANES surveys since the early 1960s and you see a disturbing trend:

Age (years)[1]	NHANES	NHANES	NHANES	NHANES	NHANES
	1963-65 1966-70[2]	1971-74	1976-80	1988-94	1999-2002
6-11	4%	4%	7%	11%	16%
12-19	5%	6%	5%	11%	16%

[1]Excludes pregnant women starting with 1971–74. Pregnancy status not available for 1963–65 and 1966–70.
[2]Data for 1963–65 is for children 6–11 years of age; data for 1966–70 is for adolescents 12–17 years of age, not 12–19 years

The 1999–2002 survey, for example, shows a 45 percent increase in overweight kids since the previous 1988–94 survey. Compare that survey to numbers from the 1960s, and there's a staggering 400 percent increase in the percentage of overweight kids (from 4 percent to 16 percent) in just four decades.

Even those numbers may be low. The American Obesity Association (AOA) reported that approximately 30.3 percent of children ages six to eleven are overweight, and 15.3 percent are classified as obese.[3] One measure of how far the problem has evolved was highlighted by a 2006 study by Johns Hopkins. It reported that, based on national growth charts as well as the 2000 Census, at least 283,305 children ages one to six are considered too heavy for standard safety seats in automobiles. For one- to three-year-olds, for example, manufacturers typically design age-specific safety harnesses for weights up to forty pounds. Yet more and more kids are now weighing more than that. These kids are not tall enough for the booster seats recommended for older children, yet they're judged to be too large for the safety seats designed for their age groups.[4] The problem is not expected to go away soon—and it is spreading beyond the U.S. According to a report published by the *International Journal of Pediatric Obesity,* nearly half of the children in North and South America will be overweight by 2010,[5] up from what recent studies say is about one-third. Our children could belong to the first generation that will grow up more obese than their parents.

What's especially alarming is that excess weight in childhood or adolescence is a good predictor of weight problems as an adult. Obese children have a greater likelihood of coming down with diseases such as type 2 adult-onset diabetes. They are prime candidates for high blood pressure, strokes, cancer, and heart disease. There's a long list of other health dangers facing kids with weight problems, including:

- High cholesterol

- Sleep apnea

- Orthopedic problems

- Liver disease

- Asthma

- Hip problems

Not least of the problems facing overweight kids is the social discrimination that comes as they interact with their peers. They are frequent targets of teasing and hazing, which in turn can lead to low self-esteem and depression.

What is causing these problems with our kids? For starters, they're eating too much and exercising too little. Researchers tell us almost half of all kids eight to sixteen years old are watching three to five hours of television a day. With computer games, the problem is compounded even more. The bottom line is that the more TV kids watch or the more computer games they play, the more likely they are to have weight problems.

So what can you do about it? Pay close attention to what is happening in your child's world. Is your child heavier than he or she should be?

Look up weight comparison charts on the Internet to see what health professionals recommend for your child at his present age. Is your child above the recommended weight levels? How much exercise is your child engaging in each day? How much food is he consuming—large portions or small? How many cold or iced drinks, especially soda, does your child consume in a day? Teenagers get 8 to 15 percent of their daily calories from carbonated and non-carbonated soft drinks. Soda provides the average twelve- to nineteen-year-old boy with approximately fifteen teaspoons of refined sugars a day, while the average girl consumes about ten teaspoons a day. This equals the government's recommended limits for a teen's daily sugar consumption from *all* foods.[6]

Consider what all that sugar—and all that ice—has been doing to your child's health. Is it any wonder, just from soda drinks alone, that kids are gaining weight? How many times a day does your child eat? Is breakfast her largest meal—or is it the meal she most often skips? How much snacking does she do? Does she snack on healthy foods such as fruits or vegetables, or does she prefer junk food? Do you keep healthy snack foods available? (Or do you expect her to find a healthy snack in a vending machine or convenience store? Good luck with that!)

How much exercise does your child get a day? Is she already a couch potato? Does she spend more than a couple of hours a day in front of a computer or television?

Incidentally, don't forget that there can be medical reasons why your child is putting on weight, especially if the weight gain is relatively quick. Certain medical conditions tend to add pounds. Ask your pediatrician for advice and counsel.

What else can you do? Plenty. Remember, however, that obesity develops over a long period of time, and the solution will not necessarily be a quick one. Treating your child's problems with weight will take time, but the time to begin is now. Prevention is always the preferred way to go—but that assumes your family has healthy habits, something fewer and fewer families can lay claim to. Incidentally, your child's weight problem is not just his or her problem—it belongs to your entire family. The whole family should be involved in the solution.

As soon your physician has checked the child and found him clear of medical problems (other than his excess weight), you may want to start your child on the Hot Diet. Considering the addiction kids have today for ice-cold sodas, this may be no mean feat. It will be no easier for your child to stop his icy drinking and eating habits than it is for you.

But unless your child—especially if a teenager—understands how his current diet and lifestyle are contributing to his weight problems, your chances of success are slim unless you explain why the Hot Diet works. Take time to demonstrate to the child how his lifestyle contributes to his condition. Paint him a picture of a life of physical ailments and dangers unless he changes his ways immediately.

Lead him through the Hot Diet, one principle at a time.

HOT DIET PRINCIPLE #1: EAT A BALANCED DIET

Kids have an endless variety of poor eating habits, but skipping meals is usually one of the most common. They learned this bad habit from us, their parents. On the positive side, they will also learn good habits from us. So when you start preaching the benefits of the Hot Diet to them, practice what you preach. Make sensible eating a family project, even for the trimmest person in the family. Your kids will do as you do, so do it right.

Teens in particular have embraced the idea of skipping breakfast as a method of weight control. "Look at all the calories we saved," they'll tell you as they struggle to squeeze into their too-tight jeans. As a begrudging response to your pleas, they might grab an energy bar or glass of juice on the way out the door.

Instead of loading up with nutritious fuel for the day ahead, they start the day on empty. An hour later, they're ravenously hungry. So they hit the vending machines in the school cafeteria. If you've seen the typical school vending machine, you know there's very little of redeeming nutritional value in many of them. Candy bars and sodas are poor replacements for a balanced breakfast.

The truth is, we've allowed our kids to become too busy for breakfast. We as a nation started putting on weight just about the time we stopped having leisurely breakfasts. We only have time to be fat these days.

Make it a house rule that from now on, breakfast is the largest meal of the day. No exceptions. If you think you can't trust yourself to enforce that rule, look at your child's expanding waistline again. How much overweight does your child have to be before you take action? If your child shows no signs of being overweight yet still skips breakfasts or other meals, will you wait for the first signs of obesity before you lay down the rule?

If you're serious about controlling your child's weight and preventing all the illnesses that can come from it, make the decision that in your house tossing down a cold glass of juice or substituting a small snack for breakfast is no longer tolerated.

Make the rule and stick to it.

Start paying closer attention to what your child eats. Serve breakfasts that consist of a healthy balance of the major food groups. Calories matter, so be aware of the number of calories your kids are consuming versus the nutritional value derived. Processed foods and sugar contain "empty" calories. Stick to the government's food pyramid, and go easy on red meat, breads, and dairy products as the pyramid suggests.

Need more ideas?

Set achievable goals for changes in your child's diet. One week set breakfast attendance as a goal. The next week, eliminate excessive snacks and sweets. Then set a goal of meeting recommended daily servings of fruits and vegetables, and so on. Use rewards when your child meets the goals—but don't make the reward something they can eat. That just defeats your purposes.

If the child who previously skipped breakfast manages to eat breakfast seven days a week, for example, treat him and a friend to a movie at the mall. If he cuts out snacks for a specified length of time, let him stay up an hour or two later on weekends. Kids respond well to incentives, so let your imagination run wild!

If your child is a fussy eater, let her choose alternate foods from the food groups. Make it his choice, but make it fun. Keep things calm and nonconfrontational. Yelling at your child to eat the meal you serve him when he cannot tolerate the taste does nothing but add to the negative energy around your breakfast table. Do yourself and your child a favor: have healthy alternatives available.

Don't be afraid to explain why you're emphasizing certain foods or eating practices. Explain, for example, how eating breakfast affects their entire day. Show them how their choices and actions can directly affect their weight, and give them your complete support in their efforts. Kids often understand more than we give them credit for, so don't be afraid to explain how the digestive system works when a large meal is consumed, and how the body needs the energy from that meal throughout the day.

Use the fire analogy, and demonstrate how fires fed by very little fuel—as in substituting a glass of juice for energy-rich food—soon burn out. The sugar in the juice gives a quick jolt of energy but quickly fizzles out. Hours, if not minutes later, the body is hungry again and working at half efficiency or less.

Help your child recognize body signals that the stomach is full. Make him aware that when he no longer feels hungry, he has the option of stopping. Never order your child to "clean your plate" just to get rid of leftover food.

Encourage your child to keep a record of his food intake. For adolescents, try making a colorful bulletin board in your kitchen. Have the child track all the times he meets his goals for meals, food consumed, and even the amount of exercise on any given day. Review the board with your child frequently, and compliment him profusely when he earns it.

In the morning, your child's body is like an eager machine. After a night's rest, it is now preparing for a full day of activity. Food is the only fuel that will keep it running at maximum efficiency. Without food, your child has no fuel; without fuel, he has no energy. Without energy, he reaches for the nearest food—usually something very convenient and typically low in nutrition—to give him a lift. Most of the time, any lift achieved is temporary.

When energy is lacking, kids do what they can to avoid activities that used to burn off fat for previous generations. Instead of walking or biking to work, they ride in the family automobile. Instead of running out to play after school, they closet themselves in their rooms with a computer or television.

Skipping breakfast—or any meal, for that matter—is a dead-end decision. Kids might get away with it for a while, but it will eventually leave its mark on their waists, thighs, and elsewhere. There's no avoiding it.

I had gone through all of this with my son, and I can't tell you how much resistance he gave me in the beginning. But eventually, after explaining again and again why his weight was ballooning beyond where it should be, I got him to the point where he agreed to at least try the Hot Diet.

In just three months, John had reached the recommended weight for his age and was looking healthier than he had in several years. He even stopped using his computer long enough to join the school football team. How did John get on board—and enthusiastic about a diet program?

PARENT TIP #1

Don't arbitrarily dictate to your child that he or she must eat breakfast, and a healthy one at that. Take the route of explaining that while breakfast is mandatory at your house, there's a good reason for it. Spend time to tell him what that reason is. (Not sure what it is? Revisit other chapters in this book!) Get the child on board intellectually, assuming he's old enough to comprehend. If he still resists, decide who the parent is. The parent rules.

PARENT TIP #2

Make breakfast not only the largest meal of the day but also the most fun and inviting. Keep the atmosphere light, positive, and enjoyable. Follow breakfast with a light lunch and a lighter dinner. Explain to your child how this structure helps him convert food to energy at times when his body needs it most.

PARENT TIP #3

Provide healthy snacks throughout the day. Substitute natural foods like fruit and vegetables for the processed foods and packaged snacks kids typically reach for. Understand that the body needs food approximately every two to three hours, so encourage healthy snacks served with hot chocolate or cider.

PARENT TIP #4

Consider adding a fourth, very light meal to the day. Children are constantly growing, so it's not surprising that they have a need for more constant conversion of food to energy than adults. Experiment with this, but don't end a four-meal day with more total calories consumed than on a three-meal day. That just adds to your problems. Try having a light meal when the kids get home from school, then another light meal a couple of hours later.

PARENT TIP #5

Avoid all foods after 8:00 p.m. Declare the refrigerator off-limits after that time with no exceptions.

PARENT TIP #6

Declare bedrooms off-limits to foods or snacks of all types at all times. This will help end "secret snacking" or "impulse snacking." Make the family dining room table or kitchen the center of all eating activities again, just as it was decades ago, and make sure your kids honor your decision.

PARENT TIP #7

Turn off the television at mealtimes. Watching TV during a meal tends to encourage mindless consumption, increases stress levels, and loses the body's "full" signals amid the distractions of on-screen excitement.

PARENT TIP #8

Become acquainted with the food and beverages offered at your school cafeteria. A few schools around the country have started to take soda machines out of the lunch area and are substituting machines with fruit drinks or milk. Under a program sponsored by former President Bill Clinton's private foundation, drink distributors have agreed to offer public high schools only diet soda, whereas elementary and middle schools will be sold only unsweetened juice, low-fat milk, and water.[7] That is definitely a step in the right direction.

Now all we have to do is take out the snack machines full of candies and other low-nutrition foods and replace them with healthier snacks. Find out where your child's school stands on vending machines and nutrition. Does the school place a higher value on the nutritional needs of its students or the revenue needs of the school? Unhealthy foods tend to cost more and generate more income for the school as compared to healthy foods. Which are offered at your school? Do you need to get more involved with other concerned parents on this issue?

Bottom line: ensure that your child has healthy food options both at school and at home. Don't buy it when kids tell you that skipping breakfast is a method of weight control. "Look at all the calories we saved," they'll tell you. It's nothing but a mini-fast, and no child should be fasting in that way. What most kids don't think about is that several hours later, with nothing in their stomachs all day, they will eat excessively for lunch or dinner, or will hit the convenience store or fast-food place for foods loaded with calories and short on nutrition.

HOT DIET PRINCIPLE #2: EAT IN MODERATION

Plain and simple, most kids eat too fast. At the same time, they eat too much. I call this the *fast-food disease* because it came into popularity at about the same time as fast-food restaurants. Slow down. You can't force the digestive system to process food faster than it was designed to do. If you try, you're just adding to excess body fat.

Your child needs to understand that dumping large amounts of food into his stomach too quickly means that the natural digestive process does not get the time it needs to function normally. If the child wolfs down his hamburger without chewing it properly, the saliva does not get a chance to begin the digestive process. Food arrives in the stomach in larger chunks and takes longer to digest. The brain does not get a chance to read the chemical signals that enough food has been consumed—the child still feels hungry. So he continues to eat.

Remember your mother or grandmother telling you to chew your food eighteen times or so before swallowing? She knew what she was talking about.

With kids, portion size is especially important. If the first words out of your child's mouth when he rushes into a restaurant are "Super size!" don't be surprised if the child is soon looking as large as his portions.

When you serve properly proportioned meals for optimum Hot Diet efficiency (large breakfast, light lunch, lighter dinner, minimal snacks as needed), kids can be trained away from the large portion habit. The Hot Diet gives your child a more manageable appetite during the day, so he is more content with smaller meals late in the day. Some friends of mine couldn't understand how this could possibly be true.

"My kid is growing so fast he's absolutely got to have twice the food of a normal person," one friend told me. "You don't understand, AJ, no kid's going to voluntarily settle for smaller portions."

I smiled and told him that my son used to eat almost constantly all day long. But when my wife and I aligned his portion sizes to what his digestive system actually needed and could efficiently handle, making sure he had food in the right portions at the most optimum times, his appetite came under control.

Control portion sizes, avoid super-sized servings, permit healthy snacks as needed, and your child will soon consume only as much food as he really needs.

HOT DIET PRINCIPLE #3: MINIMIZE STRESS

Stress throws a cold splash of water on your child's digestive system. Food eaten during stress is harder to digest, with more waste going to fat than to energy. The more peace you can introduce into your child's life, particularly at mealtimes, the better.

What are some of the ways you can help your child become less stressed? Start by making sure that your concern over her weight problem isn't making the stress worse. If you suddenly begin to make radical new rules about her diet or activity habits, you could quickly spike her stress and scuttle any programs you have for reducing her weight.

Your child wants to get rid of her weight problem as much as you do—or more—so enlist her into the planning. Focus not only on the negative aspects of behavioral change, but also on the positive benefits. Don't just dictate her path to health; nurture her on her way. If she falls off the wagon, help her back on. If she becomes discouraged, find new ways to keep her optimistic. Build her self-esteem with every pound she loses.

In all ways, promote calm during meals. Start each meal with a quiet prayer of thanksgiving. Encourage your child to lead the prayer. Outlaw family quarrels during meals. No criticism. No sarcasm. No negative comments. Enjoy the food, and be thankful for the cook.

Make your table a No-Stress Zone. If you eat with music playing in the background, make it soothing music—let your child select her favorites according to your parameters. Cancel all other activities during meals: no cell phones, no television, no interruptions from neighbors, no loud noises or drama.

Promote the enjoyment of quiet times with each other. After a meal, you and your child can experience the joy of just being in each other's company—sitting on the back patio together, gazing up at the stars, walking around the block. Talk quietly with each other. Remind yourselves of what makes you happy, and share your dreams and expectations. Tell your child a story, and ask her to tell you one in return. Rediscover the grand art of family conversation. Create pleasant memories right there on your patio.

Be a low-stress family, and your child will benefit from it.

HOT DIET PRINCIPLE #4: EXERCISE

Not many decades ago, kids came dashing home from school only to run off to the neighborhood ballpark or playground. If there were no organized sports going on, pickup games were common in every neighborhood. The average child of the 1960s exercised far more than the average child today. The exceptions these days, of course, are kids involved in school sports, other team sports, and other physical activities. But those usually aren't the kids with weight problems.

We've got to tear our kids away from televisions, computers, handheld games, video games, and the snacks they mindlessly munch on as they play. Just as any campfire quickly dies out when you fail to stoke it, no child can efficiently burn calories if he doesn't exercise and keep his muscles healthy and strong.

Begin by placing limitations on the amount of time the child can watch television or play electronic games on a daily basis. The more overweight your child is the less time you should allow for inactive entertainment.

I can guarantee you that your child will not voluntarily reduce his time with the television or electronic games. So you've got to set the standard. What will it be? One hour a day? Two? How about half of what he does now?

Once your child is off the couch and on his feet, find ways for him to get his exercise. Walking is a great start. Does your child really need a ride to school, or would a walk to school work even better (in your opinion, not your child's)? If he absolutely does need a ride, why not drop him off a few blocks from the school itself? Encourage him to walk for the sheer enjoyment of it.

Incidentally, do you really need to drive him to soccer practice or to his friend's house? Could he walk or ride a bike instead? Sometimes we parents let our children use us as taxi services more than they should.

Should you require him to participate in a school sport—even when he doesn't want to? Absolutely! You must keep the fire stirred up, and unless you get your child moving, the odds of his staying trim are small. Only if there is a physical reason—a "note from the doctor" type of thing—should your child not be engaged in school sports. Swimming, track, ball teams, and tennis are just some of the school-sponsored events that are not only fun but also offer tremendous health benefits to every participant.

Create a house rule that your child has to be outside during daylight hours. Why let him slouch in front of his computer or television when the weather is perfect for outdoor activity?

Encourage him to find some friends and start a game, go for a bike ride, or walk to a nearby park.

The Hot Diet requires some form of physical activity every day, even if only in small amounts in the beginning. The more your child exercises, the more energy he feels and the more enthusiastically he participates.

Six months ago I would never have believed my son would actually be excited to be on the school football team. But you should see him now. He's at practice three times a week, and that's three nights when he spends very little time in front of his computer!

HOT DIET PRINCIPLE #5: AVOID ICE

If you continue to permit your child to consume icy drinks, your child's weight-loss program is undoubtedly doomed to failure. Turning up the heat—getting on the Hot Diet—ensures that balanced food intake, portion control, stress control, and increased exercise are effective for more than just a few weeks. Start by getting rid of the ice in your child's diet.

Remember that even if your child were to exercise daily and eat sensibly but still had icy beverages with his food, he would continue to put on weight over many months until the excess weight is obvious to all who see him. One day you look around and suddenly wonder why tight belts run in the family.

Decide today, along with your child, that tall glasses of ice cubes and soda will no longer be served with meals in your home. Instead, start providing warm beverages such as tea or hot chocolate. Instead of cold drinks from the vending machine for school lunch, encourage your child to search for a hot alternative. Or lacking that, consider sending your child to school with a thermos of tea, hot chocolate, cider, or other warm beverage.

Don't neglect water. Encourage your child to drink at least eight glasses of water per day. While you're pouring your child's drink, don't forget that you need just as much water as he does. But it should never be ice water. Serve water at room temperature.

But what do you say to your teen who plays on the school football team and wants cold ice water in the heat of the game? Tell him to have a cool—but not cold—drink and to enjoy. Just don't have the drink with food. That's when ice has a clearly negative effect on your digestive system. So if food is involved, never drink a cold beverage with it. If no food is involved, cold beverages are OK.

The longer I practice the Hot Diet, the less I can tolerate a cold drink with my meals. That sensation of cold liquid pouring into my nice warm stomach and setting me up for weight gain is downright unpleasant. Others who have started to live the Hot Diet report the same reaction to cold drinks. Nothing compares to the long lasting, satisfying feeling that comes with a warm drink. Cold drinks lose their attraction, and slowly but surely the pounds drop off and waistlines become smaller.

With so much at stake, do not put off your child's weight control program. Start today. In summary:

- Ensure that your child's weight gain is the result of his eating habits, not a health problem. See your child's physician and follow his advice.

- Engage your child as part of the solution. Make it a joint project in which he actively participates.

- Explain in terms the child can understand how the digestive system reacts to cold and how consuming cold beverages and foods are contributing to the weight problem.

- Explain the importance of exercise in burning calories, and discuss what happens when those calories are not burned off.

- Eliminate ice drinks with meals.

- Provide healthy snack foods.

- Make a healthy, full breakfast mandatory, not optional.

- Serve light lunches and lighter dinners.

- Profusely praise all progress as the pounds melt away.

You face a challenging task as you work to get your child's weight under control. But do not let the problem become worse than it is now. Be proactive. Start your child on the Hot Diet immediately.

What parent who loves his child could possibly fail to do this?

8: QUESTIONS AND ANSWERS

Question: Do I really need to avoid ice? Can't I lose weight by simply trimming portion sizes, reducing my caloric intake, and getting plenty of daily exercise?

Answer: It's true that at first you will achieve weight loss simply by cutting down your portion sizes, reducing caloric intake, and exercising regularly. That's why so many of the diets on the market today are successful in stripping off a few pounds during the first few weeks.

Unfortunately, most of us who try fad diets gain back any weight we lose. Why? Because every one of them is based upon the misconception that food is the sole culprit. So these fad diets eliminate certain food groups—be it protein, carbohydrates, or sweets. That works for a while, but then we get bored, or we experience cravings for the foods we have given up. With the Hot Diet, you don't give up your favorite foods. You don't go hungry.

As mentioned in Chapter Three, a 2004 study by the Health and Social Care Information Centre in England showed that in spite of the fact that Britons were exercising more, the obesity rate actually doubled.[1] Exercise alone is not a good long-term solution.

The reason you should give up ice is because of its negative effect on the digestive process. By numbing the parietal cells in your stomach, the hydrochloric acid so essential for breaking down food bonds is released more slowly than when no ice is consumed. The shock of those icy cold temperatures launches a chain of events that includes using much-needed energy to raise your body temperature back to normal, encouraging the formation of fat cells as a defense against the cold and reducing the efficiency of the metabolic process. In these circumstances, food passes from the stomach and large intestinal tract to your smaller intestinal tract before it can be completely converted to energy. With less energy, you're less inclined to exercise or move about, and that in turn results in the conversion of excess calories to fat cells and the gradual loss of muscle mass.

Question: If the body expends energy rewarming the stomach when ice is introduced, wouldn't an ice diet be a good way to lose weight? Answer: The problem is that as you rewarm the body back to its normal body temperature, you are using energy you need for vital activities. So when you're ready for exercise, the energy is just not there in the amounts it should be. In addition, as discussed before, eating lots of ice tends to increase fat cells. So you will inevitably gain weight.

Question: Many times I get up in the middle of the night feeling hungry. Then, as if I have no control over myself, I go to the refrigerator and eat something cold. Lately the scale has been showing a few extra pounds. How do I control middle-of-the-night hungers?

Answer: Studies have shown that night hunger is often only thirst masquerading as hunger, so make sure you are drinking plenty of water during the day. The next time you wake up feeling hungry, have a glass of water instead of food. That should stop the hunger pangs. If, in spite of drinking more water and eating lighter dinners, you still wake up, why not use that time as an opportunity for prayer and meditation? If stress is causing your sleeplessness, then that is an excellent way to eliminate it.

Think about all the good things God has created for your loved ones and you. Focus on how grateful you are for everything around you and what a good day tomorrow is going to be. Then close your eyes and feel the love of the Creator who has taken care of you during the past years, and you will feel a calm and happy feeling and soon go back to sleep.

Question: When I go to a restaurant, I feel I have to finish the food on my plate because I have paid for it, then I feel bad that I stuffed myself. What should I do?

Answer: The fact that you have paid for the food on your plate is not a good excuse to stuff yourself. Ask for a doggie bag and take the remainder of your food home. You can always give it to a homeless person so that another human being does not go hungry. Try starting your meal with a light appetizer—and warm drink, of course—before ordering the main entrée. You won't feel so hungry because of the appetizer, and you will find yourself more content to order a smaller meal.

Eat very slowly and enjoy every bite. Chew it at least fifteen times and be grateful for the food, and as soon as your body tells you it has had enough, put down your fork. Learn to recognize the feeling of fullness, and remember that since there is sometimes a delay in that feeling, stop before you feel it. Think in terms of keeping portions to a fraction of what you're used to. The warm drink will help ensure that you feel satisfied afterward, without the stuffed feeling.

Question: What do you think about fasting? Is there any benefit?
Answer: Fasting is a method of detoxifying the body. Please consult your physician before starting any kind of fast, and when you have received approval, begin with only small periods of fasting, such as a fast from certain foods or for a single day. Be sure you drink plenty of water throughout the day. Do not use fasting to regulate weight. If you fast for religious reasons, do not go entirely without food during the day (unless your religion requires otherwise), but consider eating a small amount of bread to keep your digestive system active.

Question: How much should I eat?
Answer: Listen to your body. Your body will tell you when you are full. Follow the Hot Diet recommendations in previous chapters, eating very slowly and peacefully, chewing every bite,

and thinking good thoughts as you eat. How much we should eat is different for each of us. Each body is uniquely designed, with different requirements for energy. So a football player or runner, for example, needs more energy than a person who sits at a desk all day.

If you're six feet five inches tall, you need more food than a person who is only five feet two inches. Likewise, the type of job you have and the activities you engage in during the day will affect your food needs. A construction worker needs more food (and calories) than a computer operator.

If you want to properly align your food intake to match your individual needs, a good place to begin is by challenging your conceptions about how much food you need at your three or four main meals. Make sure breakfast is your largest meal of the day. If you are hungry between meals, have a healthy snack of fruit or vegetables. At dinner, in particular, keep portion sizes to approximately half of what you may have previously consumed.

If you accompany the food with a warm beverage, and assuming that you had a proper Hot Diet breakfast, you will be amazed at how satisfied you will be with much smaller portion sizes. Do not neglect that warm beverage, or you may feel hunger pangs! Likewise, do not neglect your daily exercise. It's a must!

Question: I want to stop consuming ice with my drinks but am finding it very difficult. Am I addicted?
Answer: It is more likely that what you're experiencing is a bad habit rather than an addiction. Your admission that you cannot

eliminate your ice consumption is a sign that (1) you recognize you have a problem, and (2) you realize you should do something about it. Experts say we can kick almost any habit in twenty-eight days. The important thing is that you begin. Naturally it may be difficult for a few days, but soon you will find that you do not even miss the ice.

In fact, I find that I am so used to not having it, that on those rare occasions when I eat or drink something cold, it is actually an unpleasant experience. I am so used to living hot that I feel the cold food or beverage as it travels all the way down my throat into my stomach, and it is not a comfortable feeling. So keep trying to rid yourself of this habit. Don't forget your water: at least eight glasses at room temperature every day. Then start cooking some of my delicious recipes, and be thankful for the opportunity to take care of your body.

Question: Why should I worry about being overweight? My dad was overweight, and he lived to be seventy-two years old before he died from his third heart attack.
Answer: It is a known fact that weight problems can decrease your life expectancy. In fact, numerous studies on rats showed that reducing their food intake actually increased their life span, sometimes by as much as 2.5 times the life spans of those that were overfed.[1]

Your father's seventy-two years are not considered a long life by today's standards. He may have lived much longer if his weight had been within recommended levels. You might live into your eighties or nineties. Keeping your weight under control means you can do more physically, avoid many of the diseases associated with excess weight, and be able to enjoy your family and friends much longer than if your weight were out of control. If you won't control your weight for yourself, how about doing it for your family?

Question: I would like to have a big, healthy breakfast. But by the time I wake up, dress, and take care of the kids, time is so short I settle for either something on the run or no breakfast at all. What's the solution?

Answer: Try waking up thirty minutes earlier. (Make sure you get the recommended eight hours of sleep per night, however.) Rising earlier is not as hard as you might think, and millions of people are discovering that getting up earlier gives them extra time they never knew they had—time for a proper breakfast. If you think that's impossible, think back to what time your parents or grandparents rose every day. Chances are it was a lot earlier than your own schedule today.

None of us is allotted more than twenty-four hours a day, so invest your allotted hours wisely—like in yourself, perhaps. Remember that you are the most important person in the world when it comes to your own personal health. There's only one *you*, and you absolutely need a nutritional breakfast. Start your day with gratitude for the time you are being given. Many people no longer have that time. Greet the morning with the attitude that you will have the best day ever, and in order to harvest all the opportunities that await you, commit yourself to giving your body the essential fuel it needs. Ask God to be with you, and be aware that He is spending the day with you.

THE HOT DIET

Question: I eat exactly the opposite of what you are recommending. As an executive at a major company, I enjoy both my success and the perks that come with it. I eat big lunches and dinners because the company pays for them. Lately I have noticed I'm gaining weight and becoming borderline obese. But hey, the food is free, as are the margaritas, iced tea, and cold beers. What should I do?

Answer: First, just say no to all those iced drinks, including iced tea. Substitute warm beverages such as tea (green tea is my favorite), hot chocolate, or caffeine-free coffee. You will see a difference in about a week. In approximately ten days, you will discover you don't need as much food. And as your weight decreases you will feel better. I have seen many executives die at a young age. How often do you hear about the forty-five-year-old guy who suddenly and unexpectedly dropped dead? And how often was that person overweight?

At executive lunches there is no law that says you have to order large, calorie-rich entrées. There's no law that says you have to have a cold salad instead of hot soup; nothing that requires you to have a beverage in a glass teeming with ice. Your employers have made an investment in you. How do you think they would react to your decision to start taking care of your weight? All the company CEOs, managers, and directors I know would love you for it.

Question: When I eat at a restaurant, the salad is so cold sometimes that I think I am getting brain freeze. How do I tell them to give me a salad that is not so cold?

Answer: Who says you have to start your meal with a salad? If it is too cold, set it aside until it warms to room temperature.

Request a warm drink or hot bowl of soup instead. Then you can eat your salad with your main entrée or after you have finished the meal. Remember, you need the roughage! The French often eat their salads last and seem to find it perfectly satisfactory. Why couldn't you do the same?

Question: How do I live the Hot Diet in the middle of summer?
Answer: Warmer weather should not be an obstacle at all. When you feel overheated due to ambient temperatures or from exercising, always cool your body from the outside, not the inside. Do not drink ice cold beverages in an attempt to cool yourself off. Instead, wear lighter clothing or shed layers. Best of all, take a cold shower. Stay hydrated. Drink at least eight glasses of water at room temperature or even a little cooler, but never with ice. Also, we recommend that you eat lots of watery fruits such as watermelon. This way you actually drink more water and will perspire, which rids your body of harmful toxins.

Question: I have already lost ten pounds on this diet. I am worried that the weight loss is only temporary. Will I gain weight back on the Hot Diet as I have on other diets?
Answer: As long as you continue to avoid icy drinks and food, exercise regularly, and follow the other Hot Diet principles, you should have no worry about gaining the weight back. Remember, worry and fear can change the chemistry of your body, so don't waste precious time and energy worrying about your weight. Instead, enjoy your life, exercise, and drink plenty of water because, as I mentioned before, the chemical reactions of digestion require plenty of water.

Question: Why should I not eat processed food?

Answer: Processed foods often seem attractive because of their convenience. It's nice to grab something out of a box without having to prepare it. But these products are often loaded with unhealthy amounts of salt or sugar (and often both) and contain lower levels of nutrients than fresh, unprocessed foods. Try some of the easy-to-make foods in our recipe section, eat plenty of fruits and vegetables, and you won't miss processed foods at all.

Question: Are potatoes or french fries bad for me?

Answer: Studies have shown that potatoes in and of themselves are not "bad." In fact, they are one of nature's "jewels," teeming with invaluable nutrients. Just one medium-sized potato gives you a good selection of the recommended daily requirements of many important vitamins and minerals. French fries, on the other hand, are potatoes cooked in trans fat and saturated fats that may be linked to obesity and heart diseases. If you love potatoes, we suggest you try boiled, baked, or mashed potatoes. And sweet potatoes are a nutritious alternative to white potatoes.

9: THE 28-DAY HOT START

So you've decided to take control of your weight. Congratulations! This is often the hardest step of all, and you should be proud of your decision to make balanced meals and sensible dieting a part of your short- and long-term health program.

Again, as recommended previously, consult with your physician and receive his approval before proceeding.

As you begin the initial phase of this diet, make sure you also commit to the other parts of the Hot Diet program: well-balanced meals, portion control and moderation, minimal stress, exercise, and avoidance of icy drinks with your meals.

We call the menus on the next few pages our 28-Day Hot Start program because it is the perfect beginning to a Hot Diet commitment that should last the rest of your life. These menus can give you a quick jump on weight loss. Many people can expect to lose ten pounds or more during the first four weeks.

Tip: a warm beverage with each of these Hot Start meals will help you keep hunger pangs to a minimum. Many people experienced no hunger at all and felt completely satisfied even with these small portions as long as they were drinking something hot along with the food.

After you have followed these menus for at least four weeks—minimizing stress at meals, making sure to exercise, and avoiding icy drinks—you can then graduate to a Hot Diet maintenance program consisting of slightly larger portion sizes.

If you're on the maintenance program and discover you need to lose a few pounds, simply go back to the 28-Day Hot Start for a few days or weeks until you lose the unwanted pounds.

But what if you go through the entire four weeks of the 28-Day Hot Start and feel you still need to lose more weight? You have two choices: You can repeat the 28-Day Hot Start, but we don't recommend repeating it more than once. Or you can begin eating the slightly larger portions of the maintenance diet and continue losing weight gradually during the next few months until you achieve your optimum weight level.

Again, we suggest you lose no more than 10 pounds a month. If you need to lose 50 pounds, take five months. If you need to lose 120 pounds, take a year.

If you still need to lose weight after the four weeks (and most of us will), you may repeat this menu, but we recommend you not do it for more than eight weeks total—and again, follow the advice of your physician. If you do not want to repeat it, continue with the Hot Diet regimen of balanced meals as recommended by the USDA's MyPyramid, moderate portion sizes, stress control, regular exercise, and no icy beverages with your food. Make some type of weight lifting part of your regular program in order to build muscle mass.

The meals in this chapter are light breakfast, light lunch, and light dinner for a full four weeks. As previously mentioned, don't be surprised if you lose ten pounds almost without effort as you follow this diet. Amazingly, the vast majority of people experience very little hunger on the 28-Day Hot Start. If you do feel hungry, simply have a small snack of fruits or vegetables.

Use the charts after each day's menu to track your progress. A monthly chart is also provided at the end of this chapter.

Enjoy!

DAY 1

Breakfast:

1 slice of whole wheat bread | omelet (2 eggs) | 1 glass of milk | 1 glass of orange juice | 1 cup of tea or coffee (decaffeinated or regular), no sugar

Snack:

1 orange

Lunch:

3-oz. lean steak | 1 small salad (room temperature) | 1 warm beverage (tea, coffee, or hot chocolate)

Snack:

4 carrot sticks

Dinner:

1 medium bowl of chicken soup (slice of whole wheat

bread or 4 crackers, optional) | 1 glass of water and a
warm beverage

Dessert:

1 slice of warm apple pie | 1 glass of warm milk

PROGRESS CHART

My weight today: _____ lbs. Minutes of exercise: _____min.

I am feeling: _____

DAY 2

Breakfast:

1 bagel with 1 tablespoon of peanut butter | 1 glass of
orange juice | 1 cup of tea or coffee (decaffeinated or
regular), no sugar

Snack:

1 tangerine and a warm beverage

Lunch:

6-oz. grilled salmon | 1 cup of cooked vegetables | 1 glass of
apple juice or a warm beverage

Snack:

4 celery sticks

Dinner:

1 medium bowl of cooked, whole wheat spaghetti with
olive oil, sautéd garlic, salt, and pepper to taste | 1 glass of
pomegranate juice | 1 small salad (room temperature) |
1 warm beverage

Dessert:

1 medium bowl of mixed fruits

PROGRESS CHART

My weight today: _____ lbs. Minutes of exercise: _____ min.

I am feeling: _____

DAY 3

Breakfast:

> 2 whole grain pancakes with 2 tablespoons of honey |
> 1 glass of orange juice | 1 glass of milk | 1 cup of tea or
> coffee (decaffeinated or regular), no sugar

Snack:

> 1 apple

Lunch:

> 6-in. grilled chicken sandwich with lettuce and tomato, no
> mayonnaise | 1 glass of V8 or grape juice | 1 warm beverage

Snack:

> 1 small yogurt, plain or with fruit

Dinner:

> 1 slice of vegetarian pizza | 2 glasses of water | 1 warm
> beverage

Dessert:

> 1 small serving of chocolate mousse | 1 glass of milk

PROGRESS CHART

My weight today: _____ lbs. Minutes of exercise: _____ min.

I am feeling: _____

DAY 4

Breakfast:

> 1 medium bowl of oatmeal | 1 glass of orange juice |

1 glass of milk | 1 cup of tea or coffee (decaffeinated or regular), no sugar

Snack:

4 medium-size dried apricots

Lunch:

1 avocado sandwich with lettuce and tomato, no mayonaise | 1 glass of V8 or grape juice

Snack:

1 small can of mixed fruits in its own juices

Dinner:

1 medium bowl of vegetable soup | 1 warm beverage

Dessert:

1 or 2 cookies | 1 cup of hot tea

PROGRESS CHART

My weight today: _____ lbs. Minutes of exercise: _____min.

I am feeling: _____

DAY 5

Breakfast:

2 whole grain waffles (with 2 tablespoons of honey) | 1 glass of orange juice | 1 glass of milk | 1 cup of tea or coffee (decaffeinated or regular), no sugar

Snack:

1 cup of grapes

Lunch:

6-oz. grilled trout | 1 small salad (room temperature) | slice of lightly buttered whole wheat bread

Snack:

   1 handful of raw almonds

Dinner:

   2 slices grilled eggplant | 1 small salad (room temperature) | slice of whole wheat bread | 1 glass of water or grape juice | 1 warm beverage

Dessert:

   5 strawberries

PROGRESS CHART

My weight today: _____ lbs. Minutes of exercise: _____ min.

I am feeling: _____

DAY 6

Breakfast:

   1 egg—any style | slice of whole wheat bread | 1 glass of orange juice | 1 glass of milk | 1 cup of tea or coffee (decaffeinated or regular), no sugar

Snack:

   1 handful of figs (dried or regular)

Lunch:

   1 beef (3-oz.) fajita with 1 cup of cooked vegetables | 1 small salad (room temperature) | 1 warm beverage

Snack:

   4 carrot or celery sticks or 1 cup of broccoli with spinach dip (made with yogurt, not mayonnaise)

Dinner:

   1 each small Idaho and sweet potato with 1 cup cooked

vegetables | 1 glass of pomegranate juice, optional |
1 warm beverage

Dessert:

1 handful of dates | 1 cup of hot tea

PROGRESS CHART

My weight today: _____ lbs. Minutes of exercise: _____ min.

I am feeling: _____

DAY 7

Breakfast:

2 slices of whole wheat toast with 2 tablespoons of honey |
1 glass of grapefruit or orange juice | 1 glass of milk | 1 cup
of tea or coffee (decaffeinated or regular), no sugar

Snack:

1 banana

Lunch:

6-in. turkey sandwich with lettuce, tomato, onion, and no
mayonnaise | 1 glass of apple juice

Snack:

1 handful of raw walnuts

Dinner:

1 medium bowl of Spanish rice with steamed broccoli and
corn | 3 glasses of water | 1 warm beverage

Dessert:

1 small serving of cherry cobbler | 1 cup of hot tea

PROGRESS CHART

My weight today: _____ lbs. Minutes of exercise: _____ min.

I am feeling: _____

DAY 8

Breakfast:

   1 slice of French toast with 1 tablespoon of honey | 1 glass of orange juice | 1 glass of milk | 1 cup of tea or coffee (decaffeinated or regular), no sugar

Snack:

   1 orange

Lunch:

   6-oz. baked cod | 1 small salad (room temperature) | 2 glasses of water

Snack:

   2 slices of cheese and 4 crackers

Dinner:

   1 medium bowl of tomato soup | 1 grilled cheese sandwich | 1 warm beverage

Dessert:

   1 piece of dark chocolate | 1 glass of warm milk

PROGRESS CHART

My weight today: _____ lbs. Minutes of exercise: _____min.

I am feeling: _____

DAY 9

Breakfast:

   spinach omelet (2 eggs) | 1 glass of orange juice | 1 glass of milk | 1 cup of tea or coffee (decaffeinated or regular), no sugar

Snack:

   2 graham crackers

Lunch:

   6-in. roast beef sandwich | 1 small salad (room temperature)

Snack:

   1 orange

Dinner:

   1 small serving of squash and zucchini casserole | 3 glasses
   of water | 1 warm beverage

Dessert:

   1 slice of lemon meringue pie | 1 cup of hot tea

PROGRESS CHART

My weight today: _____ lbs. Minutes of exercise: _____min.

I am feeling: _____

DAY 10

Breakfast:

   1 medium bowl of oatmeal | 1 glass of orange juice |
   1 glass of milk | 1 cup of tea or coffee (decaffeinated or
   regular), no sugar

Snack:

   1 handful of unsalted mixed nuts (cashews, peanuts,
   almonds, pecans, walnuts, and so on)

Lunch:

   2 pieces of chicken (baked or grilled) | 1 small salad (room
   temperature) | 1 glass of V8 or grape juice

Snack:

   mozzarella cheese with a slice of tomato on a cracker

Dinner:

   2 avocado tacos | 3 glasses of water | 1 warm beverage

Dessert:

    1 cup of mixed berries

PROGRESS CHART

My weight today: _____ lbs. Minutes of exercise: _____min.

I am feeling: _____

DAY 11

Breakfast:

    2 whole wheat English muffins (with 2 tablespoons of honey) | 1 glass of orange juice | 1 glass of milk | 1 cup of tea or coffee (decaffeinated or regular), no sugar

Snack:

    1 granola bar

Lunch:

    6-in. tuna sandwich with lettuce and tomato, no mayonnaise | 2 glasses of water

Snack:

    5 strawberries

Dinner:

    1 small eggplant stuffed with rice and tomato | 1 glass of grape juice or water

Dessert:

    1 small serving of custard | 1 cup of warm milk

PROGRESS CHART

My weight today: _____ lbs. Minutes of exercise: _____min.

I am feeling: _____

DAY 12

Breakfast:

2 eggs—any style | 1 glass of orange juice | 1 glass of milk |
1 cup of tea or coffee (decaffeinated or regular), no sugar

Snack:

1 orange

Lunch:

3-oz. pork chops | 1 small salad (room temperature)

Snack:

1 cup of plums

Dinner:

2 tablespoons of hummus with 1 pita bread | 1 small salad
(room temperature) | 1 warm beverage

Dessert:

1 slice of warm pumpkin pie

PROGRESS CHART

My weight today: _____ lbs. Minutes of exercise: _____min.

I am feeling: _____

DAY 13

Breakfast:

2 whole grain waffles with 2 tablespoons of honey | 1 glass
of orange juice | 1 glass of milk | 1 cup of tea or coffee
(decaffeinated or regular), no sugar

Snack:

4 carrot sticks

Lunch:

3-oz. grilled veal | 1 small salad (room temperature)

Snack:

4 pineapple slices

Dinner:

1 cup of grilled vegetables with olive oil and garlic powder to taste | slice of whole wheat bread | 1 warm beverage

Dessert:

1 cup of hot tea

PROGRESS CHART

My weight today: _____ lbs. Minutes of exercise: _____min.
I am feeling: _____

DAY 14

Breakfast:

1 blueberry muffin | 1 glass of orange juice | 1 glass of milk | 1 cup of tea or coffee (decaffeinated or regular), no sugar

Snack:

1 cup of grapes

Lunch:

6-in. turkey sandwich with lettuce, tomato, onion, and no mayonnaise | 1glass of apple juice

Snack:

1 handful of raw pistachios

Dinner:

1 medium bowl of fried rice and vegetables | 1 warm beverage

Dessert:

1 small plate of Jello | 1 glass of pomegranate juice

PROGRESS CHART

My weight today: _____ lbs. Minutes of exercise: _____ min.

I am feeling: _____

DAY 15

Breakfast:

slice of lightly buttered whole wheat bread | omelet
(2 eggs) | 1 glass of milk | 1 glass of orange juice | 1 cup of
tea or coffee (decaffeinated or regular), no sugar

Snack:

1 orange

Lunch:

3-oz. lean steak | 1 small salad (room temperature) |
1 warm beverage

Snack:

4 carrot sticks

Dinner:

1 medium bowl of chicken soup (slice of whole wheat
bread or 4 crackers, optional) | 1 glass of water or a warm
beverage

Dessert:

1 slice of warm apple pie | 1 glass of warm milk

PROGRESS CHART

My weight today: _____ lbs. Minutes of exercise: _____ min.

I am feeling: _____

DAY 16

Breakfast:

1 bagel with 1 tablespoon of peanut butter | 1 glass of

orange juice | 1 cup of tea or coffee (decaffeinated or regular), no sugar

Snack:

1 tangerine and a warm beverage

Lunch:

6-oz. grilled salmon | 1 cup of cooked vegetables | 1 glass of apple juice or a warm beverage

Snack:

4 celery sticks

Dinner:

1 medium bowl of cooked, whole wheat spaghetti with olive oil, sautéd garlic, and salt and pepper to taste | 1 glass of pomegranate juice | 1 small salad (room temperature) | 1 warm beverage

Dessert:

1 medium bowl of mixed fruits

PROGRESS CHART

My weight today: _____ lbs. Minutes of exercise: _____ min.

I am feeling: _____

DAY 17

Breakfast:

2 whole grain pancakes with 2 tablespoons of honey | 1 glass of orange juice | 1 glass of milk | 1 cup of tea or coffee (decaffeinated or regular), no sugar

Snack:

1 apple

Lunch:

6-in. grilled chicken sandwich with lettuce and tomato, no

mayonnaise | 1 glass of V8 or grape juice | 1 warm beverage

Snack:

1 small yogurt, plain or with fruit

Dinner:

1 slice of vegetarian pizza | 2 glasses of water | 1 warm beverage

Dessert:

1 small serving of chocolate mousse | 1 glass of milk

PROGRESS CHART

My weight today: _____ lbs. Minutes of exercise: _____min.

I am feeling: _____

DAY 18

Breakfast:

1 medium bowl of oatmeal | 1 glass of orange juice | 1 glass of milk | 1 cup of tea or coffee (decaffeinated or regular), no sugar

Snack:

4 medium-size dried apricots

Lunch:

1 avocado sandwich with lettuce and tomato, no mayonnaise | 1 glass of V8 or grape juice

Snack:

1 small can of mixed fruits in its own juices

Dinner:

1 medium bowl of vegetable soup | 1 warm beverage

Dessert:

1 or 2 cookies | 1 cup of hot tea

PROGRESS CHART

My weight today: _____ lbs. Minutes of exercise: _____ min.

I am feeling: _____

DAY 19

Breakfast:

    2 whole grain waffles (with 2 tablespoons of honey) |

    1 glass of orange juice | 1 glass of milk | 1 cup of tea or

    coffee (decaffeinated or regular), no sugar

Snack:

    1 cup of grapes

Lunch:

    6-oz. grilled trout | 1 small salad (room temperature) |

    slice of lightly buttered whole wheat bread

Snack:

    1 handful of raw almonds

Dinner:

    2 slices grilled squash or zucchini | 1 small salad (room

    temperature) | slice of whole wheat bread | 1 glass of water

    or grape juice | 1 warm beverage

Dessert:

    5 strawberries

PROGRESS CHART

My weight today: _____ lbs. Minutes of exercise: _____ min.

I am feeling: _____

DAY 20

Breakfast:

1 egg—any style | slice of whole wheat bread | 1 glass of orange juice | 1 glass of milk | 1 cup of tea or coffee (decaffeinated or regular), no sugar

Snack:

1 handful of figs (dried or regular)

Lunch:

1 vegetable fajita | 1 small salad (room temperature) | 1 warm beverage

Snack:

4 carrot or celery sticks or 1 cup of broccoli with spinach dip (made with yogurt, not mayonnaise)

Dinner:

1 each small Idaho and sweet potato with 1 cup of cooked vegetables | 1 glass of grape juice, optional | 1 warm beverage

Dessert:

1 handful of dates | 1 cup of hot tea

PROGRESS CHART

My weight today: _____ lbs. Minutes of exercise: _____min.

I am feeling: _____

DAY 21

Breakfast:

2 slices of whole wheat toast with 2 tablespoons of honey | 1 glass of grapefruit or orange juice | 1 glass of milk | 1 cup of tea or coffee (decaffeinated or regular), no sugar

Snack:

   1 banana

Lunch:

   1 avocado sandwich with lettuce and tomato, no
   mayonnaise | 1 glass of apple juice

Snack:

   1 handful of raw walnuts

Dinner:

   1 medium bowl of Spanish rice with steamed broccoli and
   corn | 3 glasses of water | 1 warm beverage

Dessert:

   1 small serving of cherry cobbler | 1 cup of hot tea

PROGRESS CHART

My weight today: _____ lbs. Minutes of exercise: _____ min.

I am feeling: _____

DAY 22

Breakfast:

   1 slice of French toast with 2 tablespoons of honey | 1 glass
   of orange juice | 1 glass of milk | 1 cup of tea or coffee
   (decaffeinated or regular), no sugar

Snack:

   1 orange

Lunch:

   6-oz. baked cod | 1 small salad (room temperature) |
   2 glasses of water

Snack:

   2 slices of cheese and 4 crackers

Dinner:

   1 medium bowl of tomato soup | 1 grilled cheese sandwich |
   1 warm beverage

Dessert:

   1 piece of dark chocolate | 1 glass of warm milk

PROGRESS CHART

My weight today: _____ lbs. Minutes of exercise: _____min.

I am feeling: _____

DAY 23

Breakfast:

   spinach omelet (2 eggs) | 1 glass of orange juice | 1 glass
   of milk | 1 cup of tea or coffee (decaffeinated or regular),
   no sugar

Snack:

   2 graham crackers

Lunch:

   6-in. roast beef sandwich | 1 small salad (room temperature)

Snack:

   1 orange

Dinner:

   1 small serving of squash and zucchini casserole | 3 glasses
   of water | 1 warm beverage

Dessert:

   1 slice of lemon meringue pie | 1 cup of hot tea

PROGRESS CHART

My weight today: _____ lbs. Minutes of exercise: _____min.

I am feeling: _____

DAY 24

Breakfast:

1 medium bowl of oatmeal | 1 glass of orange juice |
1 glass of milk | 1 cup of tea or coffee (decaffeinated
or regular), no sugar

Snack:

1 handful of unsalted mixed nuts (cashews, peanuts,
almonds, pecans, walnuts, and so on)

Lunch:

2 pieces of chicken (baked or grilled) | 1 small salad (room
temperature) | 1 glass of V8 or grape juice

Snack:

mozzarella cheese with a slice of tomato on a cracker

Dinner:

2 avocado tacos | 3 glasses of water | 1 warm beverage

Dessert:

1 cup of mixed berries

PROGRESS CHART

My weight today: _____ lbs. Minutes of exercise: _____ min.
I am feeling: _____

DAY 25

Breakfast:

2 whole wheat English muffins (with 2 tablespoons of
honey) | 1 glass of orange juice | 1 glass of milk | 1 cup of
tea or coffee (decaffeinated or regular), no sugar

Snack:

1 granola bar

Lunch:

 6-in. tuna sandwich with lettuce and tomato, no
 mayonnaise | 2 glasses of water

Snack:

 5 strawberries

Dinner:

 1 small eggplant stuffed with rice and tomato | 1 glass of
 pomegranate juice

Dessert:

 1 small serving of custard | 1 cup of warm milk

PROGRESS CHART

My weight today: _____ lbs. Minutes of exercise: _____ min.

I am feeling: _____

DAY 26

Breakfast:

 2 eggs—any style | 1 glass of orange juice | 1 glass of milk |
 1 cup of tea or coffee (decaffeinated or regular), no sugar

Snack:

 1 orange

Lunch:

 3-oz. pork chop | 1 small salad (room temperature)

Snack:

 1 cup of plums

Dinner:

 2 tablespoons hummus with 1 pita bread | 1 small salad
 (room temperature) | 1 warm beverage

Dessert:

 1 slice of warm pumpkin pie

PROGRESS CHART

My weight today: _____ lbs. Minutes of exercise: _____min.

I am feeling: _____

DAY 27

Breakfast:

2 whole grain waffles with 2 tablespoons of honey | 1 glass of orange juice | 1 glass of milk | 1 cup of tea or coffee (decaffeinated or regular), no sugar

Snack:

4 carrot sticks

Lunch:

3-oz. grilled veal | 1 small salad (room temperature)

Snack:

4 pineapple slices

Dinner:

1 cup of grilled vegetables with olive oil and garlic powder to taste | slice of whole wheat bread | 1 warm beverage

Dessert:

1 cup of hot tea

PROGRESS CHART

My weight today: _____ lbs. Minutes of exercise: _____min.

I am feeling: _____

DAY 28

Breakfast:

1 blueberry muffin | 1 glass of orange juice | 1 glass of milk | 1 cup of tea or coffee (decaffeinated or regular), no sugar

THE HOT DIET

Snack:

1 cup of grapes

Lunch:

6-in. turkey sandwich | 1 small salad (room temperature)

Snack:

1 handful of raw pistachios

Dinner:

1 medium bowl of fried rice and vegetables | 1 warm
beverage

Dessert:

1 small plate of Jello | 1 glass of grape juice

PROGRESS CHART

My weight today: _____ lbs. Minutes of exercise: _____ min.

I am feeling: _____

MONTHLY PROGRESS CHART

Track your daily weight to monitor your progress!
(Copy this page and use for future months.)

DAY	WEIGHT
1	_____
2	_____
3	_____
4	_____
5	_____
6	_____
7	_____
8	_____
9	_____
10	_____
11	_____
12	_____
13	_____
14	_____
15	_____
16	_____
17	_____

DAY	WEIGHT
18	_____
19	_____
20	_____
21	_____
22	_____
23	_____
24	_____
25	_____
26	_____
27	_____
28	_____
29	_____
30	_____
31	_____

Beginning Weight _____
Weight Today _____
Total Loss _____

10: FAVORITE
HOT DIET RECIPES

The beauty of the Hot Diet is that you have very few restrictions as to what foods or dishes you may eat and still conform to the diet. As I was researching and perfecting the Hot Diet, friends and strangers were constantly giving recipes to me. Where they got them, we don't really know.

We do know that every one of these recipes—listed here in no particular order—is absolutely delicious.

Next time you run out of ideas for what to serve for breakfast, lunch, dinner, or even snacks, reach for this list of our favorite recipes. Your whole family will love them.

The authors are not responsible for the outcome of any recipe you try from this selection. We do our best to try each one before including it in the list, but because of many variables such as different quality ingredients, temperature levels, typos, errors, omissions, or individual cooking abilities, your results may be different from ours. Remember that cooking is the art of experimentation, so if your results are less than perfect, make small changes until it comes out right.

Be adventurous. Have fun with your experiments. Enjoy!

LEMON AND PAPRIKA CHICKEN WITH RICE

Serves 6

1 whole chicken or 6 bone-in thighs	1 tablespoon olive oil
5 cups water, divided	1 large onion, chopped
Garlic powder to taste	1 leek, chopped
Lemon pepper to taste	2 tomatoes, sliced
Paprika, to taste	2 cups long-grain rice
Salt and pepper to taste	2 tomatoes, chopped
2 cups French green beans	1 cup minced fresh parsley
2 cups sliced carrots	

Remove the skin from the chicken and cut the whole chicken into pieces. In a large saucepan, bring 1 cup of the water to a boil. Add the chicken and boil for 5 minutes. Remove the chicken, reserving the broth. Place the chicken in a zip-top bag. Add garlic powder, lemon pepper, paprika, salt, and pepper to taste. Shake the bag to coat the chicken with the spices.

Steam the green beans and carrots for 5 minutes, or until tender.

In a large saucepan, heat the olive oil over medium-high heat. Add the chicken and brown on both sides. Remove the chicken and add the onion and leek and cook until translucent. Return the chicken to the pan and add the beans, carrots, the 2 sliced tomatoes, and 1 cup of the water. Cover and steam for 10 minutes.

In a medium saucepan, bring 4 cups water to a boil over medium-high heat. Add the rice and cover. Reduce the heat to medium and cook for 10 minutes, or until the rice is soft, but not fully cooked; drain.

Coat the saucepan with oil. Add half the reserved chicken broth. Return the rice to the saucepan. Add in this order the 2 chopped tomatoes, the parsley, and paprika and lemon powder to taste. Add the remaining chicken broth. Do not stir. Cover, and cook over low heat until the rice is fully cooked, about 10 minutes. Stir the rice.

Serve the rice with the chicken.

GREEN PEA SOUP

Serves 4

2 tablespoons olive oil	4 cups shelled peas
1 to 2 cups chopped onions	Salt and pepper to taste
1 leek, chopped	Chopped fresh mint to taste
5 cups chicken broth or water	2 cups fresh spinach

Heat the olive oil in a large saucepan over medium heat. Add the onions and leek and cook until tender, about 4 minutes. Add the chicken broth and peas and bring to a boil. Reduce the heat and simmer for 10 minutes or until the peas are tender. Stir in the salt, pepper, and mint.

Steam the spinach. Add to the soup. Serve and enjoy.

LENTIL SOUP

Serves 4

3 cups lentils	1 garlic clove, minced
6 to 8 cups chicken broth or water	2 bay leaves
	Ground thyme to taste
2 onions, chopped	Salt and pepper to taste

Rinse the lentils. Combine the lentils and broth in a large Dutch oven and bring to a boil over medium-high heat. Cover, reduce the heat, and simmer for 30 minutes. Add the onions, garlic, bay leaves, and thyme, salt, and pepper. Cover and simmer for 15 minutes or until thick. Discard the bay leaves. Serve with garlic bread.

VEGETABLE SOUP

Serves 4

1 tablespoon olive oil	1 tablespoon tomato paste
2 celery ribs, chopped	1 bay leaf
3 carrots, chopped	Ground thyme to taste
1 garlic clove, chopped	Dried basil to taste
2 onions, chopped	Salt and pepper to taste
4 cups water	2 zucchini, sliced
2 cups canned black-eyed	
peas, drained	

In a medium saucepan, heat the olive oil over medium-high heat. Add the celery, carrots, garlic, and onions. Sauté for 5 minutes or until tender. Add the water, black-eyed peas, tomato paste, bay leaf, and thyme, basil, salt, and pepper. Bring to a boil. Cook for 10 minutes. Add the zucchini and cook for 5 additional minutes. Remove the bay leaf before serving.

OKRA STEW

Serves 4

1 onion, chopped	1 pound okra, cut into 3 pieces
1 garlic clove, minced	1 (6-ounce) can tomato paste
1 tablespoon grapeseed oil	1 teaspoon turmeric
1 pound lean meat, cut	1 tomato, chopped
into 1-inch cubes	Salt and pepper to taste

In a large saucepan over medium-high heat, sauté the onion and garlic in the grapeseed oil until tender, about 4 minutes. Add the meat and cook for 5 minutes or until brown, stirring frequently. Add the okra, tomato paste, turmeric, tomato, and salt and pepper. Add the black-eyed peas, if preparing vegetarian stew. Add enough water to cover by 1 inch. Reduce the heat to medium and cook for 35 minutes. Serve and enjoy.

NOTE: For a vegetarian stew substitute one (15-ounce) can of black-eyed peas for the lean meat.

BEEF OR LAMB STEW

Serves 4

1 pound lean beef or lamb with
    bones, cut into 1-inch pieces

turmeric to taste

Salt and pepper to taste

Garlic powder to taste

2 onions, sliced

1 pound carrots, peeled and sliced

2 medium potatoes, peeled
    and sliced

1 (3-ounce) can tomato paste

2 cups water

Place the beef cubes in a zip-top bag. Add the turmeric, salt and pepper, and garlic powder. Shake the bag to season the meat.

In a large saucepan, place the onion slices on the bottom. Layer the seasoned beef on top of the onions. Next layer the carrots and potatoes over the beef.

In a bowl, dissolve the tomato paste in the water. Pour over the beef and vegetables. Cook over low heat, covered, for 1 hour. Serve and enjoy.

SEAFOOD SOUP

Serves 4

8 raw shrimp, peeled	1 garlic clove, chopped
8 scallops	1 tablespoon olive oil
8 clams	Salt and pepper to taste
1 medium onion, chopped	1 lemon
1 (15-ounce) can crushed tomatoes	

Rinse the shrimp, scallops, and clams. Put in a medium saucepan. Add enough water to cover. Add the onion and tomatoes and bring to a boil over medium-high heat. Cook for ten minutes.

In a skillet, heat the olive oil over medium-high heat. Add the garlic and sauté until tender. Add the garlic to the soup. Add fresh-squeezed lemon and salt and pepper to taste.

ZUCCHINI LETTUCE SALAD

Serves 4

2 heads of Romaine lettuce, chopped	1 zucchini, thinly sliced
	1 red onion, chopped
1 head of cauliflower, cut into florets	2 tablespoons extra-virgin olive oil
1 purple cabbage, chopped	2 tablespoons balsamic vinegar
10 cherry tomatoes, halved	Dried basil to taste

In a large salad bowl, combine the lettuce, cauliflower, cabbage, tomatoes, zucchini, and onion. Combine the olive oil and balsamic vinegar in a small bowl and then drizzle over the salad, tossing to coat. Sprinkle with dried basil. Serve and enjoy.

STEAK AND VEGGIE KABOBS

Serves 4

1 pound lean filet mignon	12 cherry tomatoes
2 green bell peppers	12 mushrooms
2 medium onions	Salt and pepper to taste

Cut the meat into 12 pieces. Cut each green pepper into 8 pieces. Cut each onion into 4 quarters. Thread the beef, green pepper, onion, tomato, and mushroom alternately onto each of 4 skewers. Repeat three times to make 1 kabob for each person. Place on the grill and grill to your liking. Add salt and pepper.

NOTE: Filet mignon can be substituted with one whole chicken or one pound of fresh salmon, cut into 12 pieces.

TUNA SALAD

Serves 4

1 cucumber, sliced	1 can tuna, drained
1 large tomato, chopped	1 cup fresh basil leaves, chopped
1 large onion, chopped	20 fresh mint leaves, chopped
1 garlic clove, minced	Juice of 2 limes
1 head of lettuce, chopped	2 tablespoons virgin olive oil
1 bunch spinach, chopped	1 tablespoon balsamic vinegar
(about 2 cups)	

In a bowl, combine the cucumber, tomato, onion, garlic, lettuce, spinach, tuna, basil, mint, lime juice, oil, and vinegar and mix well. Serve and enjoy.

SPINACH SALAD WITH WALNUTS AND RAISINS

Serves 2

1 bunch fresh spinach, chopped	1 cup raisins
1 medium onion, chopped	1 tablespoon extra-virgin olive oil
2 medium tomatoes, chopped	1 tablespoon balsamic vinegar
1 cucumber, sliced	Juice of 1 fresh lime or lemon
10 walnuts, halved	

In a large salad bowl, combine the spinach, onion, tomatoes, cucumber, walnuts, and raisins. Whisk together the olive oil, balsamic vinegar and lime or lemon juice in a small bowl. Pour over the salad and toss. Serve and enjoy.

STRAWBERRY SALAD

Serves 4

10 strawberries, stemmed	1 onion, chopped
1 head of lettuce, chopped	1 cup fresh basil, or
2 tomatoes, cut into 8 pieces	½ cup chopped
1 bunch fresh spinach	1 tablespoon virgin olive oil
1 (5-ounce) bag mixed salad greens	1 tablespoon balsamic vinegar
1 cucumber, peeled and sliced	2 fresh limes or lemons

In a large salad bowl, combine the strawberries, lettuce, tomatoes, spinach, mixed salad greens, cucumber, onion, and basil. In a small bowl, whisk together the olive oil, vinegar, and lime or lemon juice. Pour over the salad and toss.

FETA CHEESE, WALNUT, AND SUNFLOWER SEED SALAD

Serves 4

1 head of lettuce, chopped	10 walnuts
1 bunch fresh spinach, chopped	1 cup sunflower seeds
1 (5-ounce) bag mixed salad greens, chopped	1 cup raisins
	1 tablespoon virgin olive oil
2 tomatoes, chopped	1 tablespoon balsamic vinegar
1 cucumber, chopped	Juice of 2 fresh limes or lemons
4 ounces feta cheese crumbles	1 cup fresh basil or ½ cup chopped
1 onion, chopped	

Combine the lettuce, spinach, mixed salad greens, tomatoes, cucumber, feta cheese, onion walnuts, sunflower seeds, and raisins in a salad bowl. In a small bowl, combine the olive oil, balsamic vinegar, lime or lemon juice, and basil. Drizzle over the salad, tossing to coat. Serve and enjoy.

EGGPLANT SCRAMBLE

Serves 2

1 tablespoon olive oil or
    grapeseed oil
1 medium eggplant, cut into
    1 to 2-inch cubes
1 onion, cut into 8 pieces

½ garlic clove, minced
1 medium tomato, cut into 8 pieces
3 large eggs, beaten
Salt and pepper to taste

Heat the olive oil in a skillet over medium heat. Add the eggplant, onion, and garlic and sauté until tender. Add the tomato and cook for 1 minute. Pour in the eggs and stir for 2 to 3 minutes or until done. Add salt and pepper if desired.

MUSHROOM SCRAMBLE

Serves 1

1 tablespoon olive oil
1 green onion, chopped
6 mushrooms, quartered

1 tomato, cut into 8 pieces
2 eggs

Heat the olive oil in a skillet. Add the green onion and sauté until tender. Add the mushrooms and tomato and cook for 2 minutes. Add the eggs and cook for another 1 to 2 more minutes, stirring. Serve and enjoy.

BREAKFAST QUICHE
Mrs. Teresa Bonutto

Serves 6

2 tablespoons butter

5 eggs

¼ cup flour

½ teaspoon baking powder

1 (4-ounce) can diced green chilies

¾ cup cottage cheese

6 ounces smoked Gouda cheese, sliced

Preheat the oven to 350 degrees.

In a small bowl, melt the butter in the microwave. Beat the eggs in a medium bowl. Add the flour, baking powder, melted butter, green chilies, cottage cheese, and Gouda cheese and mix well. Pour into an 8-inch square baking dish. Bake for 35 minutes. Serve and enjoy.

APPLE–RAISIN CEREAL

Serves 3

3 apples, chopped

3 cups low-fat milk

½ teaspoon cinnamon

2 cups quick-cooking oats

½ cup chopped walnuts

1 cup raisins

Preheat the oven to 350 degrees.

In a 2-quart baking dish, combine the apples, milk, cinnamon, oats, walnuts, and raisins. Cover and bake for 15 minutes. Stir and serve.

GLORIFIED CARROTS

Mrs. N. Wilson

Serves 4

1 pound chopped cooked carrots

1 tablespoon margarine, softened

½ onion, grated

1 (10-ounce) can cream of
  mushroom soup

4 ounces Velveeta cheese

Preheat the oven to 325 degrees. Place the carrots in a 2-quart glass baking dish. Combine the margarine, onion, soup, and cheese in a bowl and mix well. Pour over the carrots. Bake, covered, for 30 minutes. Serve and enjoy.

CHOW MEIN AND ZUCCHINI CASSEROLE

Serves 5

1 medium onion, chopped

1 medium zucchini, sliced

10 mushrooms, chopped

2 cups chopped celery

1 (10-ounce) can chicken
  and rice soup

1 (15-ounce) can sliced
  water chestnuts, drained

Salt and pepper to taste

Soy sauce to taste (optional)

3 cups chow mein noodles

In a large skillet over medium-high heat, sauté the onion, zucchini, mushrooms, and celery until tender. Add the soup, water chestnuts, salt and pepper, and soy sauce if desired and mix well. Pour into 9 x 13-inch baking dish. Sprinkle the chow mein noodles evenly over the top. Bake, uncovered, for 25 minutes. Serve and enjoy.

VEGAN REUBEN SANDWICHES

Jennifer Holdt Winograd and Leslie Wilson

Makes 2 or 3 sandwiches

Thousand Island Dressing

½ cup vegan mayonnaise	½ teaspoon onion powder
½ cup ketchup	½ teaspoon salt

Sandwiches

1 tablespoon olive oil	4 to 6 rye bread slices
1 package Grand Life Seitan, sliced into 2-inch squares	1 to 1½ cups Wildwood Tofu dill salad
2 teaspoons tamari or soy sauce	⅔ to 1 cup sauerkraut
⅛ teaspoon black pepper	

For the Thousand Island dressing, combine the mayonnaise, ketchup, onion powder, and salt in a bowl and mix well. Set aside.

For the sandwiches, preheat the oven or toaster to 400 degrees. In a skillet, heat the oil over medium-high heat. Add the seitan and cook until golden brown on both sides. Sprinkle with the tamari and black pepper. Remove from the heat.

Spread the dressing on each slice of rye bread. Spread ¼ cup dill salad over half the bread slices. Top with ⅓ cup sauerkraut. Place one-third of the seitan on top of the sauerkraut. Top with 1 bread slice. Place in the oven or toaster and bake until warm. Serve and enjoy.

TURKEY TACO

Mrs. Heather Boyajian

Serves 5 to 7

1 pound ground turkey
1 (.25-ounce) package
   taco seasoning mix
1 cup salsa

¼ cup water
Marie Callender's Cornbread Mix
Olives, corn, cheese, for garnish

Preheat oven to 375 degrees. In a medium saucepan, cook the turkey until brown, stirring to crumble; drain. Add the taco seasoning mix, salsa, and water and mix well. Pour the mixture into an 11 x 8-inch baking pan. Prepare the cornbread mix as directed on the package. Pour the prepared batter on top of the turkey mixture. Bake for 25 to 30 minutes or according to the cornbread package. Serve with olives, corn, and cheese.

BBQ EGGPLANT SANDWICH

Makes 4 sandwiches

2 medium eggplants	French bread
2 tablespoons olive oil	Lettuce
Garlic powder to taste	Tomato slices
Salt and pepper to taste	Onion slices

Cut each eggplant lengthwise into four slices. Drizzle the olive oil on both sides of the eggplant slices. Season with garlic powder, salt, and pepper. Place on a grill and grill for 3 minutes on each side, or until lightly browned. Slice the French bread in half lengthwise. Place lettuce, tomato slices, onion slices, and the grilled eggplant on the bottom half of the bread. Top with the remaining half of the bread to make a very yummy sandwich. Cut into 4 sandwiches. Serve and enjoy.

GUACAMOLE DIP AND GUACAMOLE SANDWICH

Serves 4

3 ripe medium avocados, peeled and coarsely mashed	1 onion, chopped
	Juice of 2 limes or lemons
6 green olives, chopped	Garlic powder to taste
2 medium tomatoes, chopped	Salt and pepper to taste

Combine the avocado, olives, tomatoes, onion, lime juice, and garlic powder, salt, and pepper. Mix well. Serve as a dip or a spread for sandwiches.

PLAIN OR FRUIT YOGURT

Makes 4 cups

1 quart low-fat milk	4 tablespoons plain yogurt

In a medium saucepan, bring the milk to a boil over medium-low heat. Turn off the heat and let the milk cool until you can comfortably touch it with your finger. Add the yogurt and stir. Cover with a dish towel and let it sit on the counter for 8 hours or overnight. Remove the dish towel. Now you have delicious plain yogurt that you can start enjoying immediately. Add your favorite fruit, such as strawberries, blackberries, blueberries, peaches, or bananas to make fruit yogurt.

STRAWBERRY SALAD WITH
RASPBERRY VINAIGRETTE DRESSING

Jay Foersterling

Serves 6

Dressing

¾ cup sugar

¼ cup red wine vinegar

¼ cup raspberry vinegar

1 cup vegetable oil

2 garlic cloves, minced

½ teaspoon salt

½ teaspoon paprika

¼ teaspoon white pepper

Salad

2 cups Boston lettuce, torn

2 cups Romaine lettuce, torn

2 cups sliced strawberries,

1 cups shredded Muenster cheese

3 tablespoons chopped walnuts

For the dressing, in a bowl whisk together the sugar, red wine vinegar, raspberry vinegar, vegetable oil, garlic, salt, paprika, and white pepper.

For the salad, in a large bowl, combine the Boston lettuce, Romaine lettuce, strawberries, Muenster cheese, and walnuts. Pour the dressing over the salad and toss just before serving. Serve and enjoy.

FRUIT BOWL

Serves 4

3 peeled oranges, cut into sections
1 pineapple, peeled, cored, and
    cut into 1-inch pieces
2 apples, chopped

1 quart strawberries, halved
3 kiwis, peeled and sliced
1 cup raisins
1 cup yogurt, optional

In a salad bowl, combine the oranges, pineapple, apples, strawberries, kiwis, and raisins. Add yogurt on top if you desire. Serve and enjoy.

ACKNOWLEDGMENTS

I would like to express my gratitude for the efforts and kindness of thousands of people who helped with this project, but especially:

My wife and children who supported me 100 percent in this endeavor and have always been an inspiration to me.

Bill Quinn, my coauthor, who, after trying the diet and losing seventeen pounds, put in hundreds of hours and wrote tirelessly.

David Dunn, my agent, who, after trying the diet and losing fourteen pounds, encouraged me to share my revelation.

John Stoner, Peter Gluck, and Dorothy Chambers for their continuing support.

My brother and his family for being there for me.

My adopted mom, Mrs. Norma J. Wilson from Kansas.

ACKNOWLEDGMENTS

Henry Samueli for his encouraging advice to "think outside the box."

The late Senator Dewey Bartlett, who believed in humanity and education, for inviting me to Oklahoma to continue my education and giving me the chance to learn from professors such as Dr. Sam Sofer, the inventor of the artificial liver; Dr. Locke; Dr. Block; and Dr. Townsend, to name a few.

The doctors, nurses, and staff at Norris Cancer at USC, especially Dr. Robert Beart, Dr. Syma Iqbal, Dr. Emily Militzer, Yolee Casagrande, Marie Seitz, Kevin Kaneko, Thelma Ramos, and Claudia Gomez.

I am so fortunate to live in a country where I have the freedom to travel around the world to meet so many nice people who have encouraged and helped me:

John Murphy, Bob and Molly Wessel, Robin Falconer, Dr. Alfredo Sadun, Kyle Stogsdill, Craig DeYoung, Bob and Loretta Zetena, Ed and Debbie Hope, Lewis and Gayle Cohen, Dr. Lisa Major, Jessica Trucksess, Dr. Carmen Cohan, Jodi Johnson, Mark Chapman, Mathew Reil, Anna Whitmey, David Adams, Scott and Debbie Brown, John and Theresa Bonutto, Dr. Hinthorn, Dr. Maurice Borkland, Dr. Javaheri, Dr. Ruggio, Seth Brown, Paula Major, Brian Hampton, Victor Oliver, Fred Hardin, and Sonny Crews.

I am grateful that there is a library in virtually every city so I am able to read about Louis Pasteur, Albert Einstein, Sigmund Freud, Sina, Razi, and so many more.

And finally, my thanks to Sam Moore for teaching me to share knowledge that may be beneficial to others because keeping it to myself is a selfish act.

NOTES

CHAPTER ONE: THE POISON

1. 2003–2004 National Health and Nutrition Examination Survey (NHANES).

2. International Food Information Council Foundation on Obesity and Weight Management, May 2004, "Obesity and Management," www.ific.org/nutrition/obesity/index.cfm.

3. E. A. Finkelstein, I. C. Fiebelkorn, and G. Wang, "National Medical Spending Attributable to Overweight and Obesity: How Much, and Who's Paying?" *Health Affairs* 2003, W3, 219–226.

4. National Institutes of Health, www.nih.gov/news/pr/mar2005/nia-16.htm.

5. Ibid.

6. Ibid.

7. National Health and Nutrition Examination Survey, www.cdc.gov/nchs/products/pubs/pubd/hestats/ overwght99.htm.

8. Clarence Bass, "The Metabolism Myth," www.cbass.com/METABOLI.HTM.

CHAPTER TWO: THE QUEST

1. Inayat Khan and Coleman Barks, editors, *The Hand of Poetry, Five Mystic Poets of Persia* (New York: Omega Publications, 1993); Jelaludin Rumi, thirteenth-century Persian teacher and poet from Afghanistan.

2. The Journal of the American Medical Association, "Actual Causes of Death in the United States, 2000," http://jama.ama-assn.org/cgi/content/abstract/291/10/1238.

3. Abraham Lincoln, 1809–1865, sixteenth President of the U.S. www.quotationsbook.com/quotes/12389/view.

4. Lulu Hunt Peters, A.B., M.D., *Diet and Health with Key to the Calories* (Chicago: The Reilly and Lee Co., 1918); Peters was the ex-chairman of the Public Health Committee, California Federation of Women's Clubs, Los Angeles District.

CHAPTER THREE: THE DISCOVERY

1. Yair Bar David, Benjamin Gesundheit, Jacob Urkin, and Joseph Kapelushnik, "Water Intake and Cancer Prevention," *Journal of Clinical Oncology*, Vol. 22, No. 2, January 15, 2004, 383-a–385.

2. NUTRAingredients.com|europe, "Move over cola, here come health bevs," www.Nutraingredients.com/news/ ng.asp?id=38642, 19 Sep 2003.

3. Elizabeth Rosenthal, "Even the French are fighting obesity," International Herald Tribune | Europe, May 4, 2005, www.iht.com/articles/2005/05/03/news/obese.php.

4. Elaine Sciolino, "France Battles a Problem That Grows and Grows: Fat," New York Times.com, January 25, 2006.

5. Health Survey for England 2004, www.data-archive.ac.uk/doc/5439/mrdoc/pdf/5439data.pdf.

6. Ibid.

CHAPTER FOUR: LIVING HOT

1. Global Health & Fitness, "BMR Calculator," www.global-fitness.com/BMR_calc.php.

2. http://weightloss.about.com/od/eatsmart/a/b/calintake.htm.

3. Center for Disease Control and Prevention, 1998: Clinical Guidelines on the Identification, Evaluation, and Treatment of Overweight and Obesity in Adults.

4. National Library of Medicine, HSTAT, "What Is the Evidence That Obesity Has Adverse Effects on Health?" www.ncbi.nlm.nih.gov/books/bv.fcgi?rid=hstat4.section.1103.

5. International Food Information Council Foundation, "Questions and Answers About Dioxins," July 2006, www.ific.org/publications/qa/dioxinqa.cfm.

6. Harvard School of Public Health, "Food Pyramids," www.hsph.harvard.edu/nutritionsource/pyramids.html.

7. S. J. Nielsen and B. M. Popkin, "Patterns and trends in food portion sizes, 1977–1998," *Journal of the American Medical Association*, January 22, 2003; 289(4):450–453.

8. Tartamella et al., *Generation Extra Large* (NewYork: Basic Books, 2005), 61.

9. Food CPI, Prices and Expenditures: Food Away from Home, ERS-USDA, www.ers.usda.gov/Briefing/CPIFoodAndExpenditures/Data/table3.htm.

10. Hippocrates 460–359 BC, www.fnri/dost.gov.ph/wp/foodmedicine.htm.

CHAPTER FIVE: DETOUR

1. Abraham Lincoln, 1809–1865, sixteenth President of the U.S., www.quotationsbook.com/quotes/12389/view.

2. American Cancer Society Statistical Report, www.cancer.org/downloads/PRO/ColorectalCancer.pdf.

3. Ibid.

4. American Cancer Society, Signs and Symptoms of Cancer, www.cancer.org/docroot/CRI/content/CRI_2_4_3X_What_are_the_signs_and_symptoms_of_cancer.asp?sitearea.

5. www.who.int/mediacentre/factsheets/fs297/en.

6. http://ccnt.hsc.usc.edu/colorectal/newsletter3.htm.

7. American Cancer Society, "How Is Colorectal Cancer Found," www.cancer.org/docroot/CRI/content/CRI_2_2_3X_How_is_colorectal_cancer_found.asp.

CHAPTER SIX: BEYOND FOOD

1. U.S. Department of Health and Human Services, National Institutes of Health Publication No. 99-3589, Updated February 2001.

2. Chris Woolston, "The Dangers of Belly Fat," Consumer Health Interactive, Division of CareMark, March 27, 2006.

NOTES

CHAPTER SEVEN: AMERICA'S OVERWEIGHT CHILDREN

1. National Center for Health Statistics, *Trends in the Health of Americans*, 2003. Raw data source: National Health and Nutrition Examination Survey III (NHANES III), www.cdc.gov/nchs/nhanes.htm.

2. National Center for Health Statistics, *Prevalence of Overweight Among Children and Adolescents: United States, 1999–2002*, October 6, 2004.

3. American Obesity Association, *Obesity in Youth*, www.obesity.org/subs/fastfacts/obesity_youth.shtml.

4. Johns Hopkins Bloomberg School of Public Health's Center for Injury Research and Policy, "Few Child Safety Seat Models Available for Obese Children," *Pediatrics*, 3 April 2006.

5. Dr. Philip James, *International Journal of Pediatric Obesity*, March 2006.

6. Michael F. Jacobson, *Liquid Candy*, June 2005, Center for Science in the Public Interest.

7. "Alliance for a Healthier Generation—Clinton Foundation and American Heart Association—and Industry Leaders Set Healthy School Beverage Guidelines for U.S. Schools," www.clintonfoundation.org/050306-nr-cf-hs-hk-usa-pr-healthy-school-beverage-guidelines-set-for-united-states-schools.htm.

CHAPTER EIGHT: QUESTIONS AND ANSWERS

1. Health Survey for England 2004, www.data-archive.ac.uk/doc/5439/mrdoc/pdf/5439data.pdf.

2. *Anti-Aging Guide 2006*, www.anti-aging-guide.com/31mousestudies.php.